Copyright © 2021 by Elizabeth Monroe -All rights reserved.

No part of this book may be reproduced or transmitted in any form or by any means, electronic or mechanical, including photocopying and recording, or by any information storage and retrieval system, without permission in writing from the publisher. This is a work of fiction. Names, places, characters and incidents are either the product of the author's imagination or are used fictitiously, and any resemblance to any actual persons, living or dead, organizations, events or locales is entirely coincidental. The unauthorized reproduction or distribution of this copyrighted work is ilegal.

Please note the information contained within this document is for educational and entertainment purposes only. All effort has been executed to present accurate, up to date, reliable, complete information. No warranties of any kind are declared or implied. Readers acknowledge that the author is not engaged in the rendering of legal, financial, medical, or professional advice. The content within this book has been derived from various sources. Please consult a licensed professional before attempting any techniques outlined in this book. By reading this document, the reader agrees that under no circumstances is the author responsible for any losses, direct or indirect, that are incurred as a result of the use of the information contained within this document, including, but not limited to, errors, omissions, or inaccuracies.

CONTENTS

IMMUNE BOOSTING SMOOTHIES 7
- Double Decker Smoothie 7
- Papaya Passion 7
- Multi-berry Smoothie 7
- Apple-kiwi Slush 7
- Vitamin-c Boost Smoothie 7
- Flaxseed And Berry Smoothie 8
- Blueberry Peach Smoothie 8
- Popoye's Pear Smoothie For Kids 8
- Kiwi- Banana Healer 8
- Mixed Fruit Magic Smoothie 8
- Berry Carrot Smoothie 8
- Tangerine- Ginger Flu Busting Smoothie 9
- Berrilicious Chiller 9
- Strawberry-ginger Tea Smoothie 9
- Coco-maca Smoothie 9
- Banana-avocado Smoothie 9
- Berry Mint Smoothie 10
- Creamy Pink Smoothie 10
- Kiwi Cooler 10
- Orange Coco Smoothie 10
- Cacao- Spirulina And Berry Booster 10
- Pomegranate- Berry Smoothie 11
- Ultimate Cold And Flu Fighting Smoothie 11
- Citrus Spinach Immune Booster 11
- Yogi-berry Smoothie 11

DETOX AND CLEANSE SMOOTHIES 12
- Lime And Lemon Detox Punch 12
- Twisty Cucumber Honeydew 12
- Cocoa Pumpkin 12
- Dandellion- Orange Smoothie 12
- Melon-berry And Ginger Smoothie 12
- Cilantro-lemon Smoothie 13
- Green Tea- Berry Smoothie 13
- Very-berry Orange 13
- Zucchini Detox Smoothie 13
- Pear Jicama Detox Smoothie 13
- A Melon Cucumber Medley 14
- Super-detox Smoothie 14
- Carrot Detox Smoothie 14
- Honeydewmelon And Mint Blast 14
- Pineapple Coconut Detox Smoothie 14
- Blueberry Detox Drink 14
- Wheatgrass Detox Smoothie 15
- Charcoal Lemonade Detox Smoothie 15
- Avocado Detox Smoothie 15
- Tropical Smoothie 15
- Cinna-melon Detox Smoothie 15
- Apple-beet Smoothie 16
- Cacao Cantaloupe Smoothie 16
- Hearty Cucumber Quencher 16
- Coconut Pineapple Detox Smoothie 16
- Punchy Watermelon 16
- Green Grapefruit Smoothie 17
- Papaya Berry Banana Blend 17
- Apple Celery Detox Smoothie 17
- Chia Berry Cucumber Smoothie 17

PROTEIN SMOOTHIES 18
- Spiced Up Banana Shake 18
- Sweet Protein And Cherry Shake 18
- Coconut Peach Passion 18
- The Cacao Super Smoothie 18
- Strawberry Coconut Snowflake 18
- Mango Delight 18
- The Great Avocado And Almond Delight 19
- Spin-a-mango Green Protein Smoothie 19
- Peppermint And Dark Chocolate Shake Delight 19
- Iron And Protein Shake 19
- Peanut Butter Chocolate Protein Shake 19
- Honey And Cacao Bliss Smoothie 20
- Green Protein Smoothie 20
- Ginger Plum Punch 20
- Berry Orange Madness 20
- Mad Mocha Glass 20
- Protein-packed Root Beer Shake 21
- Very Creamy Green Machine 21
- Apple Mango Cucumber Crush 21
- Almond And Choco-brownie Shake 21
- Snicker Doodle Smoothie 21
- Raspberry And White Chocolate Shake 21
- Subtle Raspberry Smoothie 22
- Berry Dreamsicle Smoothie 22
- Glorious Cinnamon Roll Smoothie 22
- Maca- Almond Protein Smoothie Shake 22
- Pineapple Protein Smoothie 22
- Healthy Chocolate Milkshake 23
- Mango Mania 23
- Dark Chocolate Peppermint Smoothie 23

WEIGHT LOSS SMOOTHIES 24
- Leeks And Broccoli Cucumber Glass 24
- Spinach, Carrot And Tomato Smoothie 24
- Chia-blueberry Smoothie 24
- Healthy Raspberry And Coconut Glass 24
- Banana And Spinach Raspberry Smoothie 24
- Mint And Kale Smoothie 25
- Flax And Almond Butter Smoothie 25
- Spiced Pineapple Smoothie 25
- Zucchini Apple Smoothie 25
- A-b-c Smoothie 25
- Straight Up Avocado And Kale Smoothie 25
- Blueberry–avocado Smoothie 26
- Raspberry- Grapefruit Smoothie 26
- Banana, Almond, And Dark Chocolate Smoothie ... 26
- Pumpkin Pie Buttered Coffee 26
- Banana-mango Delight 26
- Coconutty Apple Smoothie 27
- Flax And Kiwi Spinach Smoothie 27
- Clemintine Dreamsicle Smoothie 27

Cucumber Kale And Lime Apple Smoothie 27
Peanut Butter, Banana And Cacao Smoothie .. 27
Meanie-greenie Weigh Loss Smoothie 27
Grape And Spinach Smoothie 28
Carrot Spice Smoothie 28
Veggie Wonder 28
Berry-banana-spinach Smoothie 28
Mango Strawberry Smoothie 28
Cherry-vanilla Smoothie 29
Green Tea- Mango Smoothie 29
Kale Celery Smoothie 29

KID FRIENDLY HEALTHY SMOOTHIES 30
Banana-cado Smoothie 30
Mixed Fruit Madness 30
Date Pomegranate Wonder 30
Apple Berry Smoothie 30
Pineapple Banana Smoothie 30
Peanut Butter Broccoli Smoothie 30
Berry Peachy Blush 31
The Overloaded Berry Shake 31
Kale, Cucumber Cooler 31
Pineapple Papaya Perfection Smoothie 31
Chilled Watermelon Krush 31
Mesmerizing Strawberry And Chocolate Shake 32
Very Berry Blueberry Wonder 32
Raw Chocolate Smoothie 32
Ultimate Berry Blush 32
Delish Pineapple And Coconut Milk Smoothie 32
Cool Coco-loco Cream Shake 32
Carrot Peach Blush 33
Chocolate Spinach Smoothie 33
Coconut Strawberry Punch 33
Blueberry Pineapple Blast Smoothie 33
Cocoa Banana Smoothie 33
Raspberry Pecan Date Delight 33
Delicious Creamy Choco Shake 34
Beet Berry Chiller 34
Peanut Butter Jelly Smoothie 34

HEART HEALTHY SMOOTHIES 35
Almond- Citrus Punch 35
Ginger Banana Kick 35
Berry Banana Smoothie 35
Lime And Melon Healer 35
Almond- Melon Punch 35
Chia-cacao Melon Smoothie 35
Cinn-apple Beet Smoothie 36
Almond-banana Blend 36
Spinach And Grape Smoothie 36
Mint And Avocado Smoothie 36
Peach-ban-illa Smoothie 36
Melon And Soy Smoothie 36
Mango-ginger Tango 37
Pineapple-pear And Spinach Smoothie 37
Oatmeal Banana Smoothie 37
Peach And Celery Smoothie 37
Vanilla- Mango Madness 37

Hemp-avocado Smoothie 38
Beet And Apple Smoothie 38
Pina Berry Smoothie 38
Oats And Berry Smoothie 38
Kiwi-berry-nana 38
Banana-beet Smoothie 38
Strawberry-chia Smoothie 39
Verry-berry Carrot Delight 39

OVERALL HEALTH AND WELLNESS SMOOTHIES 40
Lychee Green Smoothie 40
Pear-simmon Smoothie 40
Dragon- Berry Smoothie 40
Rasp-ricot Smoothie 40
Fruit Bomb Smoothie 40
Cherry- Date Plum Smoothie 40
Avocado- Citrus Blast 41
Yogi- Banana Agave Smoothie 41
Water-mato Green Smoothie 41
Citrus Coconut Punch 41
Blue Dragon Smoothie 41
Berry-ssimon Carrot Smoothie 41
Mp3 Smoothie 42
Date "n" Banana Smoothie 42
Red Healing Potion 42
Blueberry Cherry Wellness Potion 42
Apple Cucumber 42
Mango Cantaloupe Smoothie 43
Finana Smoothie 43
Trimelon Melba 43
Orange Cranberry Smoothie 43
Apple Blackberry Wonder 43
Drink Your Salad Smoothie 43
Chia Mango-nut Smoothie 44
Nutty Apple Smoothie 44
Peachyfig Green Smoothie 44

LOW FAT SMOOTHIES 45
Ginger Cantaloupe Detox Smoothie 45
Apple, Dried Figs And Lemon Smoothie 45
Berry-beet Watermelon Smoothie 45
Banana- Cantaloupe Wonder 45
The Pinky Swear 45
The Great Shamrock Shake 45
Chai Coconut Shake 46
The Big Blue Delight 46
Pomegranate- Ginger Melba 46
Sage Blackberry 46
A Batch Of Slimming Berries 46
Cantaloupe Berry Blast 47
Mango-berry Smoothie 47
Banana Orange Pina Colada 47
Ginger-mango Berry Blush 47
Mango Passion Smoothie 47
Pumpkin- Banana Spicy Delight 47
A Peachy Perfect Glass 48
Quick Berry Banana Smoothie 48
Slim-jim Vanilla Latte 48

Orange Banana Smoothie	48
Cauliflower Cold Glass	48
The Big Bomb Pop	49
Carrot, Watermelon And Cumin Smoothie	49
Lettuce -Orange Cooler	49
Mini Pepper Popper Smoothie	49

ANTI-AGEING SMOOTHIES ... 50

Powerful Kale And Carrot Glass	50
Beets And Berry Beauty Enhancer	50
The Anti-aging Turmeric And Coconut Delight	50
A Honeydew And Cucumber Medley	50
A Green Grape Shake	50
The Wrinkle Fighter	51
Maca – Mango Delight	51
Fine Tea Toner	51
The Feisty Goddess	51
Simple Anti-aging Cacao Dream	51
The Anti-aging Avocado	52
The Anti-aging Superfood Glass	52
The Glass Of Glowing Skin	52
4 Superfood Spice Smoothie	52
Green Tea-cacao Berry Smoothie	52
Watermelon- Yogurt Smoothie	53
The Breezy Blueberry	53
Coconut Mulberry Banana Smoothie	53
The Super Green	53
Pineapple Basil Blast	53
Dragon Fruit And Beet Smoothie	54
Mango And Blueberry Bean Smoothie	54
Date And Walnut Wonder	54
Ultimate Orange Potion	54
Cacao- Goji Berry Almond Smoothie	54
Acai Berry And Orange Smoothie	54
Natural Nectarine	55
Super Duper Berry Smoothie	55
Lychee- Cucumber Cooler	55
Apple Kale Krusher	55

DIGESTION SUPPORT SMOOTHIES ... 56

Cool Strawberry 365	56
The Baked Apple	56
Pineapple- Flax Smoothie	56
Banana Oatmeal Detox Smoothie	56
Mango-almond Smoothie	56
Beet And Pineapple Smoothie	57
Pear And Avocado Smoothie	57
Tropical Storm Glass	57
The Pumpkin Eye	57
Spin-apple Pear Smoothie	57
Noteworthy Vitamin C	57
Apple Chia Detox Smoothie	58
Basic Green Banana Smoothie	58
Blueberry Chia Smoothie	58
Pineapple Yogurt Smoothie	58
Yogurt And Plum Smoothie	58
Carrot And Prune Crunch	59
Spin-a-banana Smoothie	59

Sapodilla, Chia And Almond Milk Smoothie	59
Papaya- Mint Chiller	59
Fine Yo "mama" Matcha	59
Tomato- Melon Refreshing Smoothie	60
Mint-pineapple Cooler	60
Almond And Date Smoothie	60
Coconut Berry Smoothie	60
The Nutty Macadamia Delight	60
Hearty Papaya Drink	60
Great Green Garden	61
The Amazing Acai	61
Grape And Nectarine Blende	61

ANTI-INFLAMMATORY SMOOTHIES ... 62

Guava Berry Smoothie	62
Pineapple & Coconut Smoothie	62
Pineapple & Almond Smoothie	62
Cherry & Blueberry Smoothie	62
Cherry & Pineapple Smoothie	62
Pineapple & Mango Smoothie	62
Tangy Mango & Spinach Smoothie	63
Apple, Strawberry & Beet Smoothie	63
Pineapple, Mango & Coconut Smoothie	63
Orange Squash Tango	63
Chia And Cherry Smoothie	63
Cherry & Kale Smoothie	63
Kale & Avocado Smoothie	64
Watermelon, Berries & Avocado Smoothie	64
Cherry & Beet Smoothie	64
Mango- Papaya Blend	64
Pina-banana And Grapefruit Smoothie	64
Green Goblin Smoothie	64
Strawberry & Kale Smoothie	65
Mango-pina Smoothie	65
Ginger-carrot Punch	65
Coconut Carrot Pleasure	65
Spiced Banana Smoothie	65
Pineapple & Watermelon Smoothie	65
Blueberry & Cucumber Smoothie	66
Pear, Peach & Papaya Smoothie	66
Pineapple & Green Tea Smoothie	66
Peachy Ginger Smoothie	66
Sweet And Spicy Fruit Punch	66
Sweet Potato & Orange Smoothie	67

MUSCLE, BONE AND JOINT SMOOTHIES ... 68

Strawberry-avocado Smoothie	68
Orange Sunrise Smoothie	68
Ginger- Papaya Smoothie	68
Ginger- Parsely Grape Smoothie	68
Orange Kiwi Punch	68
Banana- Guava Smoothie	68
Apple –kiwi Blush	69
Fruit "n" Nut Smoothie	69
Kiwi Quick Smoothie	69
Ginger Lime Smoothie	69
Spinach And Kiwi Smoothie	69
Cilantro- Grapefruit Smoothie	70
Cucumber- Pineapple	70

- Pineapple Sage Smoothie 70
- Berry-cantaloupe Smoothie 70
- Orange Gold Smoothie 70
- Cucumber- Pear Healer 70
- Coconut-blueberry Smoothie 71
- Maca –banana Smoothie 71

SUPERFOOD SMOOTHIES 72
- Tea And Grape Smoothie 72
- Basil- Bee Pollen Chlorella Smoothie 72
- Aloe Vera Smoothie 72
- Berry Melon Green Smoothie 72
- Raspberry Carrot Smoothie 72
- Green Tea Superfood Smooothie 73
- Chia Berry Spinach Smoothie 73
- Blackberry Mango Crunch 73
- Oat And Walnut Berry Blast 73
- Green Chia Smoothie 73
- Hemp, Date And Chia Smoothie 74
- Nutty Mango Green Blend 74
- Choco- Berry Delight 74
- Coconut Blue Wonder 74
- Carrot Crunch Smoothie 74
- Raspberry Peach Delight 74
- Super Tropi-kale Wonder 75
- Banana-sunflower Coconut Smoothie 75
- Blue And Green Wonder 75
- Chia Flax Berry Green Smoothie 75

GREEN SMOOTHIES 76
- The Curious Raspberry And Green Shake 76
- The Coolest 5 Lettuce Green Shake 76
- Clementine Green Smoothie 76
- Banana Green Smoothie 76
- Passion Green Smoothie 76
- Berry Spinach Basil Smoothie 76
- Mango Grape Smoothie 77
- Garden Variety Green And Yogurt Delight 77
- Lovely Green Gazpacho 77
- Electrifying Green Smoothie 77
- Citrus Green Smoothie 77
- Tropical Matcha Kale 77
- Greenie Genie S Moothie 78
- The Wild Matcha Delight 78
- Dandellion Green Berry Smoothie 78
- A Mean Green Milk Shake 78
- Berry Collard Green Smoothie 78
- The Deep Green Lagoon 79
- The Minty Cucumber 79
- Date And Apricot Green Smoothie 79
- Minty Cantaloupe Smoothie 79
- The Green Potato Chai 80
- Cacao Mango Green Smoothie 80
- Blackberry Green Smoothie 80
- Tropical Apple Coconut Green Blend 80
- Lemon Cilantro Delight 80
- Cilantro And Citrus Glass 81
- Cherry Acai Berry Smoothie 81
- Pineapple And Cucumber Cooler 81
- Coco-banann Green Smoothie 81

VEGAN AND VEGETARIAN DIET SMOOTHIES 82
- Lime & Green Tea Smoothie Bowl 82
- Super Avocado Smoothie 82
- Avocado And Blueberry Smoothie 82
- Chia, Blueberry & Banana Smoothie 82
- Spinach, Grape, & Coconut Smoothie 82
- Mango, Lime & Spinach Smoothie 83
- Beet And Grapefruit Smoothie 83
- Healthy Kiwi Smoothie 83
- Green Smoothie 83
- Pina Colada Smoothie 83
- Apple, Carrot, Ginger & Fennel Smoothie 84
- Strawberry Watermelon Smoothie 84
- Caramel Banana Smoothie 84
- Raspberry Smoothie 84
- Chai Tea Smoothie 84
- Chard, Lime & Mint Smoothies 85
- Mango Smoothie 85

BRAIN HEALTH SMOOTHIES 86
- The Gritty Coffee Shake 86
- Grapefruit Spinach Smoothie 86
- Mango- Chia- Coconut Smoothie 86
- Pear 'n' Kale Smoothie 86
- Apple-papaya Medley 86
- Rosemary And Lemon Garden Smoothie 86
- Orange- Broccoli Green Monster 87
- A Whole Melon Surprise 87
- Berry Berry Smoothie 87
- Matcha Coconut Smoothie 87
- Bright Rainbow Health 87
- Berry- Green Tea Fusion Smoothie 88
- Mixed- Berry Wonder 88
- Tropical Greens Smoothie 88
- Hale 'n' Kale Banana Smoothie 88
- The Blueberry Bliss 88
- Nutty Bean "n"berry Smoothie 89
- The Wisest Watermelon Glass 89
- Berry Infusion Smoothie 89
- Mang0-soy Smoothie 89
- Pomegranate, Tangerine And Ginger Smoothie 89
- Great Nutty Lion 89
- Sweet Pea Smoothie 90
- Cacao-goji Berry Marvel 90
- Cheery Charlie Checker 90
- Cucumber Kiwi Crush 90
- 3 Spice-almond Smoothie 90
- Brain Nutrition-analyzer 91
- Cinnamon-apple Green Smoothie 91
- Apple- Blueberry Smoothie 91

BEAUTY SMOOTHIES 92
- Berry Dessert Smoothie 92
- Min-tea Mango Rejuvinating Smoothie 92
- Bluberry Cucumber Cooler 92
- Saffron Oats Smoothie 92
- Ultimate Super Food Smoothie 92

Chocolate Shake Smoothie	93
Mango-cado Blush	93
Kale And Pomegranate Smoothie	93
All In 1 Smoothie	93
Pink Grapefruit Skin	93
Pumpkin Spice Smoothie	93
Chocolaty Berry Blast	94
Pink Potion	94
Orange- Green Tonic	94
Grape And Strawberry Smoothie	94
Crunchy Kale – Chia Smoothie	94
Nutty Raspberry Avocado Blend	95
Berry Beautiful Glowing Skin Smoothie	95
Cantaloupe Yogurt Smoothie	95
Aloe Berry Smoothie	95
ENERGY BOOSTING SMOOTHIES	**96**
Pumpkin Seed And Yogurt Smoothie	96
Green Skinny Energizer	96
Avocado Wonder Smoothie	96
Orange Antioxidant Refresher	96
Persimmon Pineapple Protein Smoothie	96
Almond-banana Booster	96
Mango Honey Smoothie	97
Powerful Green Frenzy	97
Ginger- Pomegranate Smoothie	97
Berry Flax Smoothie	97
Coconut-banana Smoothie	97
Dandelion And Carrot Booster	98
Verry- Berry Breakfast	98
Apple- Date Smoothie	98
Awesome Pineapple And Carrot Blend	98
Goji Berry- Pineapple Wonder	98
Oats And Blueberry Smoothie	98
Cinnamon Mango Smoothie	99
Coco- Cranberry Smoothie	99
Banana Apple Blast	99
Generous Mango Surprise	99
Pumpkin Power Smoothie	99
Coco-nana Smoothie	100
Peppermint Stick Smoothie	100
Powerful Purple Smoothie	100
Mct Strawberry Smoothie	100
Coconut- Flaxseed Smoothie	100
Mango Beet Energy Booster	101
Mango Energizer	101
Berry- Mint Cooler	101
DIABETES SMOOTHIES	**102**
Green Tea And Carrot Smoothie	102
Hemp And Kale Smoothie	102
Cashew Apple Glass	102
Plum- Bokchoy Smoothie	102
Healthy Potato Pie Glass	102
Spicy Pear And Green Tea	103
Avocado Turmeric Smoothie	103
Tropical Kiwi Pineapple	103
Coconut Pear Crunch Smoothie	103
Cucumber-kale Chiller	103
Greens And Herbs For All	104
Diabetic Berry Blast	104
Oat, Celery Green Smoothie	104
Lime "n" Lemony Cucumber Cooler	104
Berry-licious Meta Booster	104
Peanut Butter And Raspberry Delight	105
Berry Truffle Smoothie	105
Keto Mocha Smoothie	105
Triple Berry Delight	105
Avocado And Edamame Drink	105
Cashew- Goji Berry Smoothie	105
Coconut -mint Smoothie	106
Pineapple Broccoli Smoothie	106
Cherry-berry Smoothie	106
Cacao – Avocado Smoothie	106
Strawberry – Banana Smoothie	106
Appendix : Recipes Index	**107**

IMMUNE BOOSTING SMOOTHIES

Double Decker Smoothie

Servings: 2
Cooking Time: 10 Minutes
Ingredients:
- For 1st layer (orange):
- 1 persimmon, quartered
- The juice of 1 lime
- 1 cup coconut milk
- 1 mango, peeled and chopped
- 1 tablespoon almond butter
- A pinch of cayenne pepper
- ½ teaspoon turmeric powder
- For 2nd layer (pink)
- 1 small beetroot, peeled and chopped
- 1 cup mixed berries (fresh or frozen)
- ½ cup filtered water
- 1 small grapefruit, peeled and quartered
- 5-6 fresh mint leaves
- Garnish- mint leaves, 1 teaspoon of Chia seeds

Directions:
1. Add the ingredients of the first layer into the blender and process it for 1 minute until smooth.
2. Pour the mixture equally into 2 serving glasses and keep it aside.
3. In the same blender, add the ingredients of the second layer and process whir it up until and smooth.
4. Divide this pink mixture equally into the 2 serving glass, above the first layer.
5. Sprinkle some Chia seeds on top and add a garnish with a mint leaf.
6. Serve immediately.

Nutrition Info: (Per Serving): Calories-320, Fat-5.2 g, Protein-4.5 g, Carbohydrates-72.7 g

Papaya Passion

Servings: 1
Cooking Time: 2 Minutes
Ingredients:
- 1 cup papaya, chopped
- ½ cup pineapple, peeled and chopped
- 1 cup, low fat or fat free yogurt (plain)
- 1 teaspoon coconut oil
- 1 teaspoon flaxseed powder
- A handful of ice

Directions:
1. Add the papaya, pineapple and ice into your blender and process it on medium high speed till well combined.
2. Next add the coconut oil, flaxseed powder and yogurt and process it on high speed for 1 minutes till you get a creamy, thick mixture.
3. Serve chilled!

Nutrition Info: (Per Serving): Calories-300, Fat-1.5 g, Protein- 13 g, Carbohydrates- 65 g

Multi-berry Smoothie

Servings: 1
Cooking Time: 5 Minutes
Ingredients:
- 1 cup almond/ cashew milk
- 2 blood oranges, peeled and chopped
- ½ teaspoon vanilla extract
- ½ cup mixed berries (fresh or frozen)
- ½ avocado, peeled and chopped
- ½ tablespoon cacao powder
- ½ tablespoon coconut oil

Directions:
1. Pour all the ingredients into your blender and whizz it up till the desired consistency is reached.

Nutrition Info: (Per Serving): Calories- 265, Fat-10 g, Protein- 10 g, Carbohydrates-30 g

Apple-kiwi Slush

Servings: 1
Cooking Time: 2 Minutes
Ingredients:
- 2 kiwis, peeled and chopped
- 1 apple, cored and chopped
- Cups baby spinach
- 1 large carrot, peeled and chopped
- 4 oz. filtered water

Directions:
1. Load your blender with all the ingredients and process it on high until thick and frothy.

Nutrition Info: (Per Serving). Calories-200, Fat-1.2 g, Protein- 4.8 g, Carbohydrates-51 g

Vitamin-c Boost Smoothie

Servings: 1
Cooking Time: 2 Minutes
Ingredients:
- 1 cup of pink grapefruit, peeled, deseeded and chopped
- ½ cup of strawberries (fresh or frozen)
- ½ cup pineapple, chopped
- ½ cup low fat or fat free Greek yogurt (plain)
- 2-3 ice cubes (optional)

Directions:
1. Pour all the ingredients into your blender and process until smooth.

Nutrition Info: (Per Serving): Calories- 160, Fat-0 g, Protein- 7 g, Carbohydrates- 15 g

Flaxseed And Berry Smoothie

Servings: 1
Cooking Time: 2 Minutes
Ingredients:
- 1 apple, cored and chopped
- ½ cup blueberries (fresh or frozen)
- 2 tablespoons of flaxseeds
- 1/ teaspoon of cinnamon powder
- 1/2 teaspoon of freshly squeezed lemon juice
- ¼ cup of plain fat free yogurt
- 1 teaspoon of raw organic honey
- 1 cup filtered water

Directions:
1. Place all the above ingredients into the blender jar and process until the mixture is thick and creamy.

Nutrition Info: (Per Serving): Calories- 210, Fat- 6 g, Protein- 5 g, Carbohydrates- 40 g

Blueberry Peach Smoothie

Servings: 1
Cooking Time: 5 Minutes
Ingredients:
- 1 cup almond milk
- 1 cup peach, cubed (fresh or frozen)
- A handful of blueberries (fresh or frozen)
- 1 cup greens of your choice (kale, spinach)
- 1 tablespoon of Chia seeds
- ½ teaspoon of freshly grated ginger
- 1 tablespoon of any super food of your choice
- 1 tablespoon coconut oil

Directions:
1. Add all the ingredients to the blender jar except the coconut oil and process for 1 minute.
2. Then pour in the oil and blend again for 30 seconds and serve.

Nutrition Info: (Per Serving): Calories- 280, Fat- 18 g, Protein- 3 g, Carbohydrates- 34 g

Popoye's Pear Smoothie For Kids

Servings: 1
Cooking Time: 5 Minutes
Ingredients:
- 1 pear, diced
- ½ avocado
- 1 kiwi, peeled and chopped
- A handful of baby spinach
- A few mixed berries

Directions:
1. Wash all the produce thoroughly and add them to the blender.
2. Process it for 1 minute or until well combined.
3. Serve.

Nutrition Info: (Per Serving): Calories-320, Fat-15 g, Protein-4 g, Carbohydrates-50 g

Kiwi- Banana Healer

Servings: 1
Cooking Time: 5 Minutes
Ingredients:
- 1 kiwi, peeled and chopped
- ¼ avocado, chopped
- 1 Swiss chard leaf,
- 1 small frozen banana
- 1 cup coconut water
- 1 teaspoon Spirulina powder
- 2 tablespoon hemp seeds
- 3-4 ice cubes

Directions:
1. Add all the ingredients one by one into your blender and process until smooth.

Nutrition Info: (Per Serving): Calories- 365, Fat-14 g, Protein- 11 g, carbohydrates- 47 g

Mixed Fruit Magic Smoothie

Servings: 2
Cooking Time: 2 Minutes
Ingredients:
- 1 up mixed berries (fresh or frozen)
- 1 banana, chopped (frozen)
- ½ cup fresh pineapple juice
- ½ cup fresh orange juice
- ½ cup low fat yogurt, plain

Directions:
1. Place all the ingredients listed above in the same order, one by one into your blender and whip it up on high speed until thick and creamy consistency is got.

Nutrition Info: (Per Serving): Calories-140, Fat-2.5 g, Proteins-3.5 g, Carbohydrates- 30 g

Berry Carrot Smoothie

Servings: 1
Cooking Time: 2 Minutes
Ingredients:
- ¾ cup of freshly squeezed orange juice
- ½ cup of low fat plain yogurt
- 1 small carrot, chopped

- 1 cup mixed berries (preferably frozen)
- 2 tablespoon pumpkin seeds

Directions:
1. Just add all the ingredients into your blender jar and process the smoothie until it's nice and frothy.

Nutrition Info: (Per Serving): Calories- 159, Fat- 5 g, Protein- 4 g, Carbohydrates- 25 g

Tangerine- Ginger Flu Busting Smoothie

Servings: 2 Small
Cooking Time: 2 Minutes
Ingredients:
- 5 California tangerines, peeled and chopped
- 2 cups mixed greens like kale, chard, dandelion or lettuce
- 1 banana chopped (fresh or frozen)
- 1 teaspoon freshly grated ginger
- ¼ cup filtered water

Directions:
1. Just pour all the ingredients into the blender and pulse until smooth.
2. Pour into individual serving glasses and serve.

Nutrition Info: (Per Serving): Calories- 247, Fats-1 g, Proteins-5 g, Carbohydrates- 61 g

Berrilicious Chiller

Servings: 2
Cooking Time: 5 Minutes
Ingredients:
- 1 ½ cup mixed berries (fresh or frozen)
- 1 tablespoon freshly squeezed lemon juice
- 6 ounces of unsweetened almond milk
- 2 teaspoons of freshly grated ginger
- 1 tablespoon flax seeds
- 1 ½ tablespoons of raw organic honey
- A handful of ice cubes

Directions:
1. Add all the ingredients into your blender and process until smooth and frothy.
2. Serve and enjoy immediately.

Nutrition Info: (Per Serving): Calories- 110, Fat-1.5 g, Protein- 1 g, Carbs-26 g

Strawberry-ginger Tea Smoothie

Servings: 1
Cooking Time: 5 Minutes
Ingredients:
- 1 cup freshly brewed ginger tea (warm or hot)
- ½ cup strawberries, tops removed
- 1 oranges, peeled and chopped
- ½ line, peeled and chopped
- Juice of ½ lemon
- ¼ teaspoon of freshly grated ginger
- 1 clove of garlic
- A pinch of cayenne pepper
- ¼ teaspoon of cinnamon powder
- 1 teaspoon coconut oil
- 2 tablespoons raw, organic honey
- A pinch of sea salt
- 4-5 cubes of ice (optional)

Directions:
1. Prepare a cup of ginger tea and keep it aside.
2. Add all the ingredients into your blender except the tea and process it for a minute.
3. Then add the tea and pulse it for another minute or until well blended.

Nutrition Info: (Per Serving): Calories- 210, fat- 5 g, Protein- 1 g, Carbohydrates- 50 g

Coco-maca Smoothie

Servings: 1
Cooking Time: 5 Minutes
Ingredients:
- 1 cup coconut milk,
- 1 banana (fresh or frozen)
- A handful of mixed berries
- 1 teaspoon coconut oil
- ½ teaspoon vanilla extract
- ⅓ tablespoon Cacao powder
- 1 tablespoon Chia seeds
- ½ teaspoon raw, organic honey or liquid stevia (optional)

Directions:
1. Load your blender with all the ingredients and pulse it up until there are no more lumps.

Nutrition Info: (Per Serving): Calories-285, Fat-7 g, Protein-21 g, Carbohydrates-40 g

Banana-avocado Smoothie

Servings: 1
Cooking Time: 2 Minutes
Ingredients:
- 2 kiwis, peeled and chopped
- 1 large banana, chopped
- 2 cups spinach
- 2 tablespoons avocado flesh
- A pinch of cinnamon powder
- ½ cup filtered water

Directions:
1. Fill up your blender jar with the fruits, greens, and water and blend until well combined.

2. Sprinkle a dash of cinnamon powder on top and serve.
Nutrition Info: (Per Serving): Calories-300, Fat-8.3 g, Protein- 6.3 g, Carbohydrates -60.6 g

Berry Mint Smoothie

Servings: 1
Cooking Time: 5 Minutes
Ingredients:
- 1 cup strawberries, fresh or frozen
- 1 cup unsweetened almond milk
- 2 kale leaves, chopped
- 1 tablespoon Chia seeds
- 1 tablespoon lemon zest
- 1 teaspoon raw, organic honey
- 1-2 sprigs of fresh mint
- 1-2 ice cubes (optional)

Directions:
1. To you blender, add all the above ingredient and pulse until smooth.

Creamy Pink Smoothie

Servings: 2
Cooking Time: 5 Minutes
Ingredients:
- 2 cups strawberries (fresh or frozen)
- 2 tablespoon cashew butter
- 1 ½ cup of almond milk (unsweetened)
- 2 tablespoons rolled oats
- 1 teaspoon vanilla extract
- 1 teaspoon raw organic honey
- A pinch of cinnamon power
- 1 teaspoon of cashew flakes (garnish)

Directions:
1. Place all the ingredients in your blender and run it on high for 1 minute.
2. Pour into serving glasses and top it with a sprinkle of cashew flakes.
3. Enjoy!

Kiwi Cooler

Servings: 1
Cooking Time: 2 Minutes
Ingredients:
- 2 kiwis, peeled and chopped
- 1 banana, fresh or frozen
- 2 cups greens of your choice
- 2-4 mint leaves
- 4 ounces of filtered water

Directions:

1. Add all the ingredients into your blender jar and pulse it until smooth.
Nutrition Info: (Per Serving): Calories- 223, Fat 1.2 g, Protein- 5.3 g, Carbohydrates- 56.3 g

Orange Coco Smoothie

Servings: 2
Cooking Time: 10 Minutes
Ingredients:
- 1 cup freshly squeezed orange juice
- 6 California tangerines, peeled and chopped
- 1 cup mixed greens
- 2 teaspoons freshly grated ginger root
- Juice of 2 freshly squeezed lemons
- 1 ½ cups of coconut milk/ coconut water (your choice)
- 4 teaspoons pure coconut oil
- 2 tablespoons Chia seeds
- 4 teaspoons raw organic honey
- 1 tablespoons any super food of your choice

Directions:
1. To your blender jar, add all the ingredients in the given order and whirr it up for 90 seconds or until done.
Nutrition Info: (Per Serving): Calories-267, Fat-1.3 g, Protein-5.3 g, Carbohydrates- 68.4 g

Cacao- Spirulina And Berry Booster

Servings: 1
Cooking Time: 5 Minutes
Ingredients:
- 1 banana, (fresh or frozen)
- 1 cup coconut milk
- 1 cup strawberries (fresh or frozen)
- 1 cup mixed greens
- ½ cup blueberries (frozen)
- 1 teaspoon cacao powder
- 1 teaspoon Spirulina powder
- ½ tablespoon coconut oil
- A large pinch of cinnamon powder
- 1 teaspoon of raw, organic honey,
- 1 tablespoon of any super food of your choice 9 mace, goji berry, bee pollen, aloe, hemp etc.)

Directions:
1. Load your smoothie blender with all the mentioned ingredients and pulse it on high speed for 2 minutes.
2. Pour into a glass and enjoy.
Nutrition Info: (Per Serving): Calories- 390, Fat- 18 g , Protein- 15 g, Carbohydrates- 50 g

Pomegranate- Berry Smoothie

Servings: 1
Cooking Time: 2 Minutes
Ingredients:
- ¾ cup freshly squeezed pomegranate juice
- 1 cups mixed berries (fresh or frozen)
- 1 cup low fat yogurt
- 2-3 drops of vanilla extract
- 1 teaspoon Chia seeds

Directions:
1. Add all the above ingredients into your blender jar and pulse until thick and frothy.

Nutrition Info: (Per Serving): Calories- 283, Fat-3 g, Protein-7 g, Carbohydrates-58 g

Ultimate Cold And Flu Fighting Smoothie

Servings: 1
Cooking Time: 5 Minutes
Ingredients:
- 1 large banana, fresh or frozen
- 2 oranges, peeled and chopped
- 2 cups baby spinach
- Freshly squeezed juice of ½ lemon
- 2 tablespoon Chia seeds (soaked)
- 1 teaspoon of freshly grated ginger
- ¼ cup of filtered water

Directions:
1. Whizz all the ingredients in the blender until smooth and serve.

Nutrition Info: (Per Serving): Calories- 330, Fat- 5.8 g, Protein-8 g, Carbohydrates-72 g

Citrus Spinach Immune Booster

Servings: 2
Cooking Time: 5 Minutes
Ingredients:
- 1 orange, peeled, deseeded and chopped
- 1 lime, peeled, deseeded and chopped
- A small handful of spinach leaves, washed
- 1-2 peaches, peeled and chopped
- 2 carrots, peeled and chopped
- 1 ½ cups almond milk (unsweetened)

Directions:
1. Dump all the ingredients into the blender and whip it up until the smoothie is thick and creamy.

Nutrition Info: (Per Serving): Calories-145, Fat-2g, Protein- 4 g, Carbohydrates- 30 g

Yogi-berry Smoothie

Servings: 1
Cooking Time: 5 Minutes
Ingredients:
- 2 cups mixed greens of your choice
- 1 cup pineapple, chopped
- ½ orange, peeled and chopped
- 1 kiwi, peeled and chopped
- ½ cup mixed berries (fresh or frozen)
- ½ cup low fat Greek yogurt (plain)
- 1 tablespoon flax seeds (soaked or ground)
- ½ cup filtered water

Directions:
1. To your blender, add all the smoothie ingredients listed above and process until smooth and creamy.

Nutrition Info: (Per Serving): Calories-330, Fat-3.4 g, Protein-18.4 g, Carbohydrates- 162 g

DETOX AND CLEANSE SMOOTHIES

Lime And Lemon Detox Punch

Servings: 2
Cooking Time: 5 Minutes
Ingredients:
- 1 banana, chopped (fresh or frozen)
- ½ cup blueberries (fresh or frozen)
- 1 cup fresh kale stems chopped off
- ½ sweet lime, peeled, de-seeded and chopped
- 1 tablespoon freshly squeezed Lemon juice
- ½ tablespoon freshly grated ginger
- 1 cup filtered water
- 1 teaspoon raw organic honey
- A pinch of Celtic salt

Directions:
1. Place all the ingredients into your blender and puree it on medium high until the smoothie is thick and frothy.

Nutrition Info: (Per Serving): Calories- 190, Fat- 1 g, Protein- 3 g, Carbohydrates- 51 g

Twisty Cucumber Honeydew

Servings: 2
Cooking Time: 5 Minutes
Ingredients:
- 1 cup ice
- 1 tablespoon fresh mint
- 2 cucumbers, chopped
- 1 cup honeydew melon, peeled, seeded, and chopped
- 1 cup coconut water

Directions:
1. Add all the ingredients except vegetables/fruits first
2. Blend until smooth
3. Add the vegetable/fruits
4. Blend until smooth
5. Add a few ice cubes and serve the smoothie
6. Enjoy!

Nutrition Info: Calories: 70; Fat: 1g; Carbohydrates: 13g; Protein: 2g

Cocoa Pumpkin

Servings: 2
Cooking Time: 5 Minutes
Ingredients:
- ¼ teaspoon pumpkin spice
- 1 tablespoon maple syrup
- 2 tablespoons organic unsweetened cocoa powder
- ¼ frozen banana, sliced
- ½ Barlett pear, cored
- 3 cups baby spinach
- 1 cup organic pumpkin puree
- 1 cup unsweetened almond milk

Directions:
1. Add all the ingredients except vegetables/fruits first
2. Blend until smooth
3. Add the vegetable/fruits
4. Blend until smooth
5. Add a few ice cubes and serve the smoothie
6. Enjoy!

Nutrition Info: Calories: 486; Fat: 28g; Carbohydrates: 64g; Protein: 11g

Dandellion- Orange Smoothie

Servings: 2
Cooking Time: 5 Minutes
Ingredients:
- 1 cup unsweetened almond milk
- 1 cup dandelion greens, washed and chopped
- 1 cup kale, (stems removed)
- 1 large orange, peeled and de seeded
- ½ lime, peeled and deseeded
- 1 ripe banana (fresh or frozen)
- ¼ teaspoon freshly grated ginger
- 1 tablespoon Chia seeds (soaked)
- 2-3 ice cubes

Directions:
1. Add all the ingredients to your blender and process until smooth and creamy.

Nutrition Info: (Per Serving): Calories- 320, Fat- 4 g, Protein- 9 g, Carbohydrates- 64 g

Melon-berry And Ginger Smoothie

Servings: 2
Cooking Time: 5 Minutes
Ingredients:
- 2 cups watermelon, peeled and chopped (seedless s or seeded)
- ½ cup blueberries (fresh or frozen)'
- 1 cup mixed greens
- ½ cup raspberries (fresh or frozen)
- Freshly squeezed juice of ½ lime
- A pinch of sea salt or Celtic salt
- 1 teaspoon freshly grated ginger
- A handful of ice cubes

Directions:

1. Into your blender jar, add all the above listed ingredients and pulse until the desired consistency is reached.
2. Serve chilled!

Nutrition Info: (Per Serving): Calories- 142, Fat- 1 g, Protein- 3 g, Carbohydrates- 35 g

Cilantro-lemon Smoothie

Servings: 2
Cooking Time: 5 Minutes
Ingredients:
- 1 large apple, cored and chopped
- ⅓ Fresh cilantro
- ¼ cup fresh flat leaf parsley
- 1-2 stalk of celery, chopped
- 1 cup fresh kale stems removed and chopped
- 1 tablespoon of flax seeds
- 2 tablespoon freshly squeezed lemon juice
- ¼ teaspoon cinnamon powder
- 1 ½ cups of filtered water

Directions:
1. Add all the ingredients into your blender and run it on medium high for 1 minute.
2. Pour and enjoy this delicious smoothie immediately.

Nutrition Info: (Per Serving): Calories: 190, Fat- 3 g, Protein- 5.7 g, Carbohydrates- 40 g

Green Tea- Berry Smoothie

Servings: 2
Cooking Time: 10 Minutes
Ingredients:
- 1 cup green tea (chilled)
- 1/3 cup raspberries (fresh or frozen)
- 1/3 cup blueberries (fresh or frozen)
- 1/3 cup black berries (fresh or frozen)
- ½ small avocado, peeled and chopped
- 1 cup fresh spinach, washed
- 1/3 cup plain yogurt
- 2 teaspoon of freshly squeezed lemon juice

Directions:
1. First, prepare a cup green tea as usual (sugarless) and let it cool down at room temperature.
2. Then chill it in the refrigerator for a few minutes.
3. After the tea has chilled, pour all the ingredients into the blender jar and whizz it for 1 minute or until the smoothie is thick and creamy.

Nutrition Info: (Per Serving): Calories- 365. Fat- 15 g, Protein-10 g, Carbohydrates- 56.6 g

Very-berry Orange

Servings: 1 Large
Cooking Time: 2 Minutes
Ingredients:
- 1 cup blueberries, fresh or frozen
- 1 cup raspberries, fresh or frozen
- 2 large oranges, peeled and chopped
- A few ice cubes

Directions:
1. Add everything to the blender and process on high for 30 seconds.
2. Pour into glass and serve chilled.

Nutrition Info: (Per Serving): Calories- 132, Fat-0 g, Protein- 2 g, Carbohydrates- 34 g

Zucchini Detox Smoothie

Servings: 2
Cooking Time: 10 Minutes
Ingredients:
- 1 zucchini
- 1 tablespoon sea beans
- ½ lemon, juiced
- 1 teaspoon maqui berry powder
- 8 tablespoons grape tomatoes
- 6 tablespoons celery stocks
- ½ jalapeno pepper, seeded
- 1 cup of water
- 1 cup ice

Directions:
1. Add all the listed ingredients to blender except zucchini
2. Add zucchini and blend the mixture
3. Blend until smooth
4. Serve chilled and enjoy!

Nutrition Info: Calories: 50; Fat: 0.5g; Carbohydrates: 10g; Protein: 2.4g

Pear Jicama Detox Smoothie

Servings: 2
Cooking Time: 10 Minutes
Ingredients:
- 3 tablespoons red kale
- 8 tablespoons jicama, peeled and chopped
- 1 lemon, juiced
- 1 pear, chopped
- 1 teaspoon reishi mushroom
- 1 tablespoon flaxseed
- 1 cup of water
- 1 cup ice

Directions:
1. Add all the listed ingredients to a blender
2. Blend until smooth

3. Serve chilled and enjoy!
Nutrition Info: Calories: 102; Fat: 0g; Carbohydrates: 24g; Protein: 2g

A Melon Cucumber Medley

Servings: 2
Cooking Time: 5 Minutes
Ingredients:
- ¾ cup honeydew melon, peeled and chopped
- 2 cups kale, chopped
- 1 medium cucumber, cubed

Directions:
1. Add all the ingredients except vegetables/fruits first
2. Blend until smooth
3. Add the vegetable/fruits
4. Blend until smooth
5. Add a few ice cubes and serve the smoothie
6. Enjoy!

Nutrition Info: Calories: 112; Fat: 2g; Carbohydrates: 30g; Protein: 2g

Super-detox Smoothie

Servings: 2
Cooking Time: 5 Minutes
Ingredients:
- ½ avocado, peeled, pitted and chopped
- ½ cup papaya, chopped (fresh or frozen)
- ½ cup pineapple, chopped (fresh or frozen)
- 1 cup mango, chopped (fresh or frozen)
- A handful of fresh spinach
- ½ cup cilantro, washed
- Freshly squeezed juice of 1 lime
- 1 tablespoon coconut oil
- 1 teaspoon raw, organic honey
- ½ teaspoon freshly grated ginger
- 1 teaspoon spirulina powder
- 1 cup filtered water
- A few ice cubes

Directions:
1. Add all the ingredients into your blender except the honey, oil an ice and whizz for 1 minute until nicely everything is pureed.
2. Then add the remaining ingredients and pulse on high for 30 seconds until well combined.

Nutrition Info: (Per Serving): Calories-314, Fat- 15 g, Protein- 5 g, Carbohydrates- 48 g

Carrot Detox Smoothie

Servings: 2
Cooking Time: 10 Minutes
Ingredients:
- 10 tablespoons carrot, chopped
- 1-inch ginger, peeled and chopped
- 1 teaspoon cinnamon
- 1 banana, peeled
- 1-inch turmeric peeled, chopped
- 1 cup of coconut milk
- 1 cup ice

Directions:
1. Add all the listed ingredients to a blender
2. Blend until smooth
3. Serve chilled and enjoy!

Nutrition Info: Calories: 134; Fat: 3g; Carbohydrates: 30g; Protein: 2g

Honeydewmelon And Mint Blast

Servings: 2
Cooking Time: 2 Minutes
Ingredients:
- Cup cucumber, peeled and chopped
- 1 cup honeydew melon, peeled and chopped
- 1 cup freshly squeezed pear juice
- ¼ cup freshly squeezed lime juice
- ¼ cup fresh mint leaves, washed
- 2-3 cubes of ice (optional)

Directions:
1. Place all the ingredients into your blender and puree until smooth.

Nutrition Info: (Per Serving): Calories- 134, Fat-0 g, Protein- 2 g, Carbohydrates-33 g

Pineapple Coconut Detox Smoothie

Servings: 2
Cooking Time: 10 Minutes
Ingredients:
- 4 cups kale, chopped
- 2 cups of coconut water
- 2 bananas
- 2 cups pineapple

Directions:
1. Add all the listed ingredients to a blender
2. Blend until you have a smooth and creamy texture
3. Serve chilled and enjoy!

Nutrition Info: Calories: 299; Fat: 1.1g; Carbohydrates: 71.5g; Protein: 7.9g

Blueberry Detox Drink

Servings: 2

Cooking Time: 5 Minutes
Ingredients:
- 1 cup ice
- 2 tablespoons spirulina
- ½ frozen banana, sliced
- 2 cups blueberries, frozen
- 2 cups baby spinach
- 2 cups coconut water

Directions:
1. Add all the ingredients except vegetables/fruits first
2. Blend until smooth
3. Add the vegetable/fruits
4. Blend until smooth
5. Add a few ice cubes and serve the smoothie
6. Enjoy!

Nutrition Info: Calories: 685; Fat: 60g; Carbohydrates: 40g; Protein: 32g

Wheatgrass Detox Smoothie

Servings: 2
Cooking Time: 10 Minutes
Ingredients:
- 3 tablespoons Swiss chard
- 1 banana, peeled
- 3 tablespoons almonds
- 1 teaspoon wheatgrass powder
- 2 kiwis, peeled
- 1 cup ice
- 1 cup of water

Directions:
1. Add all the listed ingredients to blender except kiwis
2. Blend until smooth
3. Add kiwis and blend again
4. Serve chilled and enjoy!

Nutrition Info: Calories: 154; Fat: 6g; Carbohydrates: 24g; Protein: 4g

Charcoal Lemonade Detox Smoothie

Servings: 2
Cooking Time: 10 Minutes
Ingredients:
- 3 tablespoons collard green
- ½ teaspoon charcoal activated
- 1 apple, chopped
- 1 lemon, peeled
- ½ inch ginger
- 1 cucumber, chopped
- 1 cup ice
- 1 cup of water

Directions:
1. Add all the listed ingredients to blender except kiwis
2. Blend until smooth
3. Add kiwis and blend again
4. Serve chilled and enjoy!

Nutrition Info: Calories: 88; Fat: 0.6g; Carbohydrates: 23g; Protein: 2g

Avocado Detox Smoothie

Servings: 3
Cooking Time: 10 Minutes
Ingredients:
- 4 cups spinach, chopped
- 1 avocado, chopped
- 3 cups apple juice
- 2 apples, unpeeled, cored and chopped

Directions:
1. Add all the listed ingredients to a blender
2. Blend until you have a smooth and creamy texture
3. Serve chilled and enjoy!

Nutrition Info: Calories: 336; Fat: 13.8g; Carbohydrates: 55.8g; Protein: 3g

Tropical Smoothie

Servings: 3
Cooking Time: 5 Minutes
Ingredients:
- ½ cup mango, chopped (fresh or frozen)
- ½ cup freshly squeezed orange juice
- 1 medium banana (fresh or frozen)
- ½ cup pineapple, chopped
- ¼ cup baby spinach
- ¼ cup kale (stems removed)
- 2 tablespoon freshly squeezed lemon juice
- 1 teaspoon pure coconut oil
- ½ teaspoon freshly grated ginger
- ½ cup filtered water
- A few ice cubes (if needed)

Directions:
1. Place all the ingredients into your blender and whirr it up on high for 1 minute or until done.

Nutrition Info: (Per Serving): Calories- 200, Fat- 5 g, Protein- 2 g, Carbohydrates- 40 g

Cinna-melon Detox Smoothie

Servings: 2-3
Cooking Time: 5 Minutes
Ingredients:
- 1 cup watermelon, chopped

- 1 cup dandelion greens, washed and chopped
- 1 large banana, fresh or frozen
- Freshly squeezed juice from ½ lime
- Freshly squeezed juice of 1 lemon
- ½ teaspoon raw organic honey (optional)
- ½ teaspoon turmeric powder
- 1 teaspoon freshly grated ginger powder
- ¼ teaspoon of cinnamon powder
- 8 ounces of filtered water
- 1-2 ice cubes

Directions:
1. Pour all the ingredients into your blender and process until thick and frothy.

Nutrition Info: (Per Serving): Calories- 182, Fat- 1 g, Protein- 4 g, Carbohydrates- 45 g

Apple-beet Smoothie

Servings: 2
Cooking Time: 5 Minutes
Ingredients:
- 1 large apple, cored and chopped
- 1 green pear, cored and chopped,
- 1 carrot, peeled and chopped
- ½ cup red beet, peeled and chopped
- 2 tablespoons freshly squeezed lemon juice
- 2 teaspoons freshly grated ginger

Directions:
1. First, steam the carrot and beets for about 10-12 minutes, until tender and allow it to cool.
2. Once it is at room temperature, add the steamed beets and carrots to the blender along with the other ingredients and pulse until smooth.

Nutrition Info: (Per Serving): Calories- 135, Fat- 0 g, Protein- 2 g, Carbohydrates- 35 g

Cacao Cantaloupe Smoothie

Servings: 2
Cooking Time: 5 Minutes
Ingredients:
- 1 cup unsweetened almond milk
- 1 cup whole strawberries (fresh or frozen)
- 1 cup cantaloupe, chopped
- 1 banana, chopped (fresh or frozen)
- 2-3 fresh chard leaves
- 1 tablespoon cacao powder
- 1 tablespoon Chia seeds, Soaked

Directions:
1. Add all the ingredients into your blender and process on medium high speed for 45 seconds or until done.

Nutrition Info: (Per Serving): Calories- 330, Fat- 0 g, Protein- 10 g, Carbohydrates- 61 g

Hearty Cucumber Quencher

Servings: 2
Cooking Time: 5 Minutes
Ingredients:
- 2 cups kale, chopped
- 1 fuji apple, quartered
- 1 large cucumber, cubed

Directions:
1. Add all the ingredients except vegetables/fruits first
2. Blend until smooth
3. Add the vegetable/fruits
4. Blend until smooth
5. Add a few ice cubes and serve the smoothie
6. Enjoy!

Nutrition Info: Calories: 180; Fat: 2g; Carbohydrates: 40g; Protein: 5g

Coconut Pineapple Detox Smoothie

Servings: 2
Cooking Time: 10 Minutes
Ingredients:
- 3 tablespoons Swiss Chard
- 2 tablespoons coconut flakes
- 1 tablespoon chia seeds
- 8 tablespoons pineapple, peeled and chopped
- ½ avocado pitted
- 1 orange, peeled
- 1 cup of water
- 1 cup ice

Directions:
1. Add all the listed ingredients to a blender
2. Blend until smooth
3. Serve chilled and enjoy!

Nutrition Info: Calories: 212; Fat: 0g; Carbohydrates: 26g; Protein: 3g

Punchy Watermelon

Servings: 2
Cooking Time: 5 Minutes
Ingredients:
- 1 large cucumber, cubed
- 1 cup kale, chopped
- 1 cup baby spinach, chopped
- 4 cups watermelon, chopped

Directions:
1. Add all the ingredients except vegetables/fruits first
2. Blend until smooth
3. Add the vegetable/fruits

4. Blend until smooth
5. Add a few ice cubes and serve the smoothie
6. Enjoy!

Nutrition Info: Calories: 464; Fat: 20g; Carbohydrates: 65g; Protein: 23g

Green Grapefruit Smoothie

Servings: 2-3
Cooking Time: 5 Minutes
Ingredients:
- 1 grapefruit, peeled, deseeded and chopped
- 1 large orange, peeled and chopped
- 2 chard leaves, washed
- 2 cups fresh mixed greens or baby spinach
- 2 cups strawberries (fresh or frozen)
- 1 large banana (fresh or frozen)
- 1 cup filtered water

Directions:
1. To your blender jar, add all the ingredients in the given order and process oh high for 1-2 minutes until smooth and thick.

Nutrition Info: (Per Serving): Calories- 345, Fat- 1 g, Protein- 7 g, Carbohydrates- 85 g

Papaya Berry Banana Blend

Servings: 2
Cooking Time: 5 Minutes
Ingredients:
- 1 cup, homemade, unsweetened almond milk
- 1 ½ cup papaya, peeled and chopped
- 1 large banana, chopped (fresh or frozen)
- A handful of fresh strawberries
- 1 large pitted peach

Directions:
1. Add the fruits and almond milk into the blender and puree until thick and creamy.

Nutrition Info: (Per Serving): Calories- 318, Fat- 3 g, Protein- 5 g, Carbohydrates- 70 g

Apple Celery Detox Smoothie

Servings: 2
Cooking Time: 10 Minutes
Ingredients:
- 3 tablespoons collard greens
- 2 ribs celery
- 3 springs mint
- 1 apple, chopped
- 2 tablespoons hazelnuts, raw
- ½ teaspoon moringa
- 1 cup of water
- 1 cup ice

Directions:
1. Add all the listed ingredients to a blender
2. Blend until you have a smooth and creamy texture
3. Serve chilled and enjoy!

Nutrition Info: Calories: 115; Fat: 5g; Carbohydrates: 14g; Protein: 3g

Chia Berry Cucumber Smoothie

Servings: 2
Cooking Time: 5 Minutes
Ingredients:
- 1 cup unsweetened almond milk
- 2 cups mixed berries (fresh or frozen)
- 1 banana, chopped
- 1 cup kale stems removed
- ½ cup flat leaf parsley, washed
- 1 large apple, cored and chopped
- ¼ cup cucumber, chopped
- Freshly squeezed juice of 1 lemon
- 1 tablespoon Chia seeds, soaked
- 1 cup filtered water

Directions:
1. Add all the ingredients to your blender and pulse on high for 1-2 minutes or until well combined.

Nutrition Info: (Per Serving): Calories- 220, Fat- 3 g, Protein- 5 g, Carbohydrates- 47 g

PROTEIN SMOOTHIES

Spiced Up Banana Shake

Servings: 2
Cooking Time: 5 Minutes
Ingredients:
- 2 scoops vanilla protein powder
- ½ teaspoon ground cinnamon
- 1/8 teaspoon ground nutmeg
- 2 ripe bananas
- 12 ice cubes

Directions:
1. Add all the ingredients except vegetables/fruits first
2. Blend until smooth
3. Add the vegetable/fruits
4. Blend until smooth
5. Add a few ice cubes and serve the smoothie
6. Enjoy!

Nutrition Info: Calories: 506; Fat: 30g; Carbohydrates: 56g; Protein: 12g

Sweet Protein And Cherry Shake

Servings: 2
Cooking Time: 5 Minutes
Ingredients:
- 1 cup water
- 3 cups spinach
- 2 bananas, sliced
- 2 cups frozen cherries
- 2 tablespoons cacao powder
- 4 tablespoons hemp seeds, shelled

Directions:
1. Add all the ingredients except vegetables/fruits first
2. Blend until smooth
3. Add the vegetable/fruits
4. Blend until smooth
5. Add a few ice cubes and serve the smoothie
6. Enjoy!

Nutrition Info: Calories: 111; Fat: 3g; Carbohydrates: 9g; Protein: 13g

Coconut Peach Passion

Servings: 3
Cooking Time: 5 Minutes
Ingredients:
- 1 cup unsweetened coconut milk
- 1 ½ cups peach, pitted and chopped
- ¾ cup plain low fat green yogurt
- ½ cup rolled oats
- 1 large ripe banana, chopped
- ¼ teaspoon vanilla extract
- ¼ cup filtered water
- 2-3 ice cubes

Directions:
1. Whizz up all the ingredients in the high speed blender until smooth and serve immediately.

Nutrition Info: (Per Serving): Calories- 265, Fat- 3.2 g, Protein- 12 g, Carbohydrates- 35 g

The Cacao Super Smoothie

Servings: 1
Cooking Time: 10 Minutes
Ingredients:
- ½ avocado, peeled, pitted, sliced
- ½ cup frozen blueberries, unsweetened
- ½ cup almond milk, vanilla, unsweetened
- ½ cup half and half
- 1 scoop whey vanilla protein powder
- 1 tablespoon cacao powder
- Liquid stevia

Directions:
1. Add listed ingredients to a blender
2. Blend until you get a smooth and creamy texture
3. Serve chilled and enjoy!

Nutrition Info: Calories: 445; Fat: 14g; Carbohydrates: 9g; Protein: 16g

Strawberry Coconut Snowflake

Servings: 2
Cooking Time: 2 Minutes
Ingredients:
- ½ unsweetened, fresh coconut milk
- 1 cup whole strawberries (fresh or frozen)
- ½ cup plain low fat Greek yogurt
- ¼ cup freshly squeezed orange
- ½ teaspoon raw organic honey
- 2-3 ice cubes

Directions:
1. Just place all the ingredients into the blender and pulse until smooth. Serve immediately!

Nutrition Info: (Per Serving): Calories- 160, Fat- 2.8 g, Protein- 12 g, Carbohydrates- 24 g

Mango Delight

Servings: 2
Cooking Time: 5 Minutes
Ingredients:
- 1 large mango, peeled and chopped
- ¾ cup low fat tofu

- ½ cup unsweetened almond milk
- ½ large banana, chopped
- ½ teaspoon honey (optional)
- 2-3 ice cubes

Directions:
1. Place all the above ingredients into the blender jar and process until the mixture is thick and creamy.

Nutrition Info: (Per Serving): Calories- 345, Fat- 10 g, Protein- 15 g, Carbohydrates- 60 g

The Great Avocado And Almond Delight

Servings: 1
Cooking Time: 10 Minutes
Ingredients:
- ½ avocado, peeled, pitted and sliced
- ½ cup almond milk, vanilla and unsweetened
- ½ teaspoon vanilla extract
- ½ cup half and half
- 1 tablespoon almond butter
- 1 scoop Zero Carb protein powder
- Pinch of cinnamon
- 2-4 ice cubes
- Liquid stevia

Directions:
1. Add all the listed ingredients into your blender
2. Blend until smooth
3. Serve chilled and enjoy!

Nutrition Info: Calories: 252; Fat: 18g; Carbohydrates: 5g; Protein: 17g

Spin-a-mango Green Protein Smoothie

Servings: 3
Cooking Time: 5 Minutes
Ingredients:
- 1 cup unsweetened almond milk
- ½ ripe banana, chopped
- ¼ cup mango, chopped
- ¼ cup pineapple, chopped
- 1 cup fresh baby spinach, washed and chopped
- 2 teaspoon flaxseeds
- 2 teaspoon chia seeds
- 1 teaspoon raw organic honey (optional)
- 2-3 ice cubes

Directions:
1. Whizz up all the above listed ingredients in your blender for 20 seconds and serve. Enjoy immediately.

Nutrition Info: (Per Serving): Calories- 240, Fat- 8 g, Protein- 20 g, Carbohydrates- 22 g

Peppermint And Dark Chocolate Shake Delight

Servings: 2
Cooking Time: 5 Minutes
Ingredients:
- ¼ teaspoon peppermint extract
- 1 scoop chocolate whey protein powder
- 2 tablespoons cocoa powder
- Pinch of salt
- 1 cup almond milk
- 1 large frozen banana
- 2-3 large ice cubes

Directions:
1. Add all the ingredients except vegetables/fruits first
2. Blend until smooth
3. Add the vegetable/fruits
4. Blend until smooth
5. Add a few ice cubes and serve the smoothie
6. Enjoy!

Nutrition Info: Calories: 374; Fat: 26g; Carbohydrates: 26g; Protein: 16g

Iron And Protein Shake

Servings: 2
Cooking Time: 5 Minutes
Ingredients:
- 2 tablespoons favorite sweetened syrup
- 1 cup water
- ¼ cup hemp seeds
- 2 large bananas, frozen
- 4 cups strawberries, sliced

Directions:
1. Add all the ingredients except vegetables/fruits first
2. Blend until smooth
3. Add the vegetable/fruits
4. Blend until smooth
5. Add a few ice cubes and serve the smoothie
6. Enjoy!

Nutrition Info: Calories: 156; Fat: 14g; Carbohydrates: 1g; Protein: 7g

Peanut Butter Chocolate Protein Shake

Servings: 3
Cooking Time: 5 Minutes
Ingredients:
- 1 cup unsweetened almond milk
- 1/2 cup rolled oats
- teaspoon vanilla extract
- 2 tablespoons powdered peanuts
- 2 tablespoons homemade peanut butter

- 2 tablespoons flaxseed powder
- 2 tablespoons raw cacao powder
- 4 egg whites, raw (liquid form)
- ¾ cup plain low fat yogurt
- 3-5 ice cubes

Directions:
1. Place all the above ingredients into the blender jar and process until the mixture is thick and creamy.

Nutrition Info: (Per Serving): Calories- 730, Fat- 21 g, Protein- 60 g, Carbohydrates- 81 g

Honey And Cacao Bliss Smoothie

Servings: 1 Large
Cooking Time: 2 Minutes
Ingredients:
- ½ cup unsweetened almond milk
- 3 teaspoons peanut butter
- 1 ripe banana, chopped
- 2 teaspoons raw cacao powder
- 1 ½ teaspoon raw organic honey
- 2-3 ice cubes

Directions:
1. To your high speed blender, add all the above mentioned items and process on high for 30 seconds. Pour into serving glasses and enjoy immediately.

Nutrition Info: (Per Serving): Calories- 440, Fat- 20 g, Protein- 13 g, Carbohydrates- 56 g

Green Protein Smoothie

Servings: 2
Cooking Time: 10 Minutes
Ingredients:
- 2 bananas
- 4 cups mixed greens
- 2 tablespoons almond butter
- 1 cup almond milk, unsweetened

Directions:
1. Add all the listed ingredients to a blender
2. Blend until you have a smooth and creamy texture
3. Serve chilled and enjoy!

Nutrition Info: Calories: 230; Fat: 5.8g; Carbohydrates: 39.5g; Protein: 7.8g

Ginger Plum Punch

Servings: 4
Cooking Time: 5 Minutes
Ingredients:
- 1 ½ cups tofu
- ½ cup unsweetened almond milk
- 1 cup whole strawberries (fresh or frozen)
- 1 cup whole raspberries (fresh or frozen)
- ¼ cup Goji berries
- ¼ cup whole almonds
- ½ teaspoon vanilla extract
- 1 teaspoon freshly grated ginger
- 1-2 teaspoons raw organic honey
- 8-10 mint leaves
- 4-5 ice cubes

Directions:
1. Place all the ingredients into the blender, secure the lid and whizz on medium high for 30 seconds or until done. Serve immediately.

Nutrition Info: (Per Serving): Calories- 240, Fat- 6.8 g, Protein- 15 g, Carbohydrates- 33g

Berry Orange Madness

Servings: 2-3
Cooking Time: 2 Minutes
Ingredients:
- 1 cup mixed berries (fresh or frozen)
- 1 large orange, peeled, seeded and segmented
- 1 cup low fat plain yogurt
- 1 banana, chopped (frozen)
- ¼ teaspoon vanilla extract
- 1-2 ice cubes

Directions:
1. Pour all the ingredients into your blender and process until smooth.

Nutrition Info: (Per Serving): Calories-210, Fat-2 g, Protein- 8.3 g, Carbohydrates- 40 g

Mad Mocha Glass

Servings: 2
Cooking Time: 5 Minutes
Ingredients:
- 4 ice cubes
- 1 scoop 100% chocolate whey protein
- ½ scoop vanilla protein powder
- 6 ounces water
- 6 ounces cold coffee

Directions:
1. Add all the ingredients except vegetables/fruits first
2. Blend until smooth
3. Add the vegetable/fruits
4. Blend until smooth
5. Add a few ice cubes and serve the smoothie
6. Enjoy!

Nutrition Info: Calories: 306; Fat: 4g; Carbohydrates: 43g; Protein: 28g

Protein-packed Root Beer Shake

Servings: 2
Cooking Time: 5 Minutes
Ingredients:
- ½ cup fat-free vanilla yogurt
- 1 scoop vanilla whey protein
- 1½ cups root beet
- 1 scoop vanilla casein protein

Directions:
1. Add all the ingredients except vegetables/fruits first
2. Blend until smooth
3. Add the vegetable/fruits
4. Blend until smooth
5. Add a few ice cubes and serve the smoothie
6. Enjoy!

Nutrition Info: Calories: 677; Fat: 56g; Carbohydrates: 39g; Protein: 16g

Very Creamy Green Machine

Servings: 1
Cooking Time: 10 Minutes
Ingredients:
- ½ cup frozen blueberries, unsweetened
- ½ avocado, peeled, pitted and sliced
- ½ cup unsweetened almond milk, vanilla
- ½ cup half and half
- 1 cup spinach
- 2-4 ice cubes
- 1 tablespoon almond butter
- 1 scoop Zero Carb protein powder
- 1 pack stevia

Directions:
1. Add listed ingredients to a blender
2. Blend until you have a smooth and creamy texture
3. Serve chilled and enjoy!

Nutrition Info: Calories: 279; Fat: 18g; Carbohydrates: 9g; Protein: 18g

Apple Mango Cucumber Crush

Servings: 3
Cooking Time: 5 Minutes
Ingredients:
- ½ cup freshly pressed red grapefruit juice
- 1 cup fresh kale, stems removed and chopped
- 1 large apple, cored and chopped
- ½ cup mango, peeled and chopped
- 1 cup English cucumber, chopped
- 1-2 small stalks of celery, chopped
- 5 teaspoons of hemp seeds
- 1 tablespoon pure coconut oil
- 3 -4 teaspoons of fresh mint leaves, chopped
- 4-5 ice cubes

Directions:
1. Add all the above listed items into the blender and blend until well combined.

Nutrition Info: (Per Serving): Calories- 265, Fat- 13 g, Protein- 10 g, Carbohydrates- 33 g

Almond And Choco-brownie Shake

Servings: 2
Cooking Time: 5 Minutes
Ingredients:
- ½ chocolate brownie bar, chopped
- ¼ cup almonds, chopped
- 1 scoop chocolate whey protein
- 1 cup fat-free milk

Directions:
1. Add all the ingredients except vegetables/fruits first
2. Blend until smooth
3. Add the vegetable/fruits
4. Blend until smooth
5. Add a few ice cubes and serve the smoothie
6. Enjoy!

Nutrition Info: Calories: 578; Fat: 35g; Carbohydrates: 69g; Protein: 17g

Snicker Doodle Smoothie

Servings: 2 Small
Cooking Time: 2 Minutes
Ingredients:
- 1 cup unsweetened almond milk
- 1 teaspoon raw, organic cacao powder
- 1/3 cup peanut butter or peanut powder
- 1 large ripe banana, chopped
- 3-5 ice cubes

Directions:
1. Whizz all the ingredients in the blender until smooth and serve.

Nutrition Info: (Per Serving): Calories- 315, Fat- 10 g, Protein- 28 g, Carbohydrates- 45 g

Raspberry And White Chocolate Shake

Servings: 2
Cooking Time: 5 Minutes
Ingredients:
- 2 scoops whey vanilla protein powder
- 1 tablespoon chia seeds
- 1 tablespoon white chocolate chips
- 2 tablespoons water

- 1 cup coconut milk, unsweetened
- ¾ cup frozen raspberries

Directions:
1. Add all the ingredients except vegetables/fruits first
2. Blend until smooth
3. Add the vegetable/fruits
4. Blend until smooth
5. Add a few ice cubes and serve the smoothie
6. Enjoy!

Nutrition Info: Calories: 574; Fat: 35g; Carbohydrates: 34g; Protein: 34g

Subtle Raspberry Smoothie

Servings: 1
Cooking Time: 10 Minutes
Ingredients:
- ½ cup raspberries
- 1 scoop vanilla whey protein powder
- 1 scoop prebiotic fiber
- 1 cup unsweetened almond milk, vanilla
- 2 tablespoons coconut oil
- ¼ cup coconut flakes, unsweetened
- 3-4 ice cubes

Directions:
1. Add all the listed ingredients into your blender
2. Blend until smooth
3. Serve chilled and enjoy!

Nutrition Info: Calories: 258; Fat: 22g; Carbohydrates: 7g; Protein: 14g

Berry Dreamsicle Smoothie

Servings: 3 - 4
Cooking Time: 5 Minutes
Ingredients:
- 1 cup whole blueberries (fresh or frozen)
- 1/2 ripe banana, chopped
- ½ cup whole strawberries (fresh or frozen)
- 3 large handfuls of chopped lucent kale
- 1 tablespoon freshly squeezed lemon juice
- 2 tablespoons chia seeds
- ½ cup filtered water
- 3-4 ice cubes

Directions:
1. Whizz all the ingredients in the blender until smooth and serve.

Nutrition Info: (Per Serving): Calories- 400, Fat- 10.5 g, Protein- 17 g, Carbohydrates- 70 g

Glorious Cinnamon Roll Smoothie

Servings: 1
Cooking Time: 10 Minutes
Ingredients:
- 1 cup unsweetened almond milk
- ½ teaspoon cinnamon
- ¼ teaspoon vanilla extract
- 1 tablespoon chia seeds
- 2 tablespoons vanilla protein powder
- 1 cup ice cubes

Directions:
1. Add all the listed ingredients into your blender
2. Blend until smooth
3. Serve chilled and enjoy!

Nutrition Info: Calories: 145; Fat: 4g; Carbohydrates: 1.6g; Protein: 0.6g

Maca- Almond Protein Smoothie Shake

Servings: 2
Cooking Time: 2 Minutes
Ingredients:
- 1 cup unsweetened almond milk
- 1 large ripe banana, chopped
- 2 teaspoons Chia seeds
- 2 teaspoons almond butter
- ½ cup baby spinach
- 1 teaspoon cacao powder
- 1 teaspoon Maca root powder
- A dash of cinnamon

Directions:
1. Add all the above ingredients into your blender jar and pulse until thick and frothy.

Nutrition Info: (Per Serving): Calories-281, Fat- 15 g, Protein- 18 g, Carbohydrates- 40 g

Pineapple Protein Smoothie

Servings: 3-4
Cooking Time: 5 Minutes
Ingredients:
- 1 ½ cups pineapple, chopped
- 1 medium ripe banana, chopped
- 1 cup plain low fat yogurt
- 1 cup plain unsweetened almond milk
- 2-3 ice cubes

Directions:
1. Place everything in the blender jar, secure the lid and pulse until smooth.

Nutrition Info: (Per Serving): Calories- 170, Fat- 4.7 g, Protein- 11 g, Carbohydrates- 25 g

Healthy Chocolate Milkshake

Servings: 2
Cooking Time: 10 Minutes
Ingredients:
- 1 Scoop Whey isolate chocolate protein powder
- 16 ounces unsweetened almond milk, vanilla
- 1 pack stevia
- ½ cup crushed ice

Directions:
1. Add all the listed ingredients to a blender
2. Blend until you have a smooth and creamy texture
3. Serve chilled and enjoy!

Nutrition Info: Calories: 292; Fat: 25g; Carbohydrates: 4g; Protein: 15g

Mango Mania

Servings: 2
Cooking Time: 2 Minutes
Ingredients:
- 1 large cup mango, peeled and chopped
- 2 teaspoons help hearts
- ¾ cup freshly prepared apple juice
- 1 tablespoons goji berries
- ½ teaspoon chili powder
- 1 tablespoon freshly squeezed lemon juice
- 1 tablespoon freshly squeezed lime juice
- ½ cup filtered water
- 1 teaspoon raw organic honey
- 2-3 ice cubes (optional)

Directions:
1. Place all the above ingredients into the blender jar and process until the mixture is thick and creamy.

Nutrition Info: (Per Serving): Calories- 325, Fat- 8 g, Protein- 6 g, Carbohydrates- 61 g

Dark Chocolate Peppermint Smoothie

Servings: 2
Cooking Time: 10 Minutes
Ingredients:
- 2 large bananas, frozen
- 2 scoops chocolate protein powder
- 4 tablespoons cocoa powder
- 2 cups almond milk
- 2 pinches sea salt
- ½ teaspoon peppermint extract
- 4 large ice cubes
- 1 tablespoon dark chocolate chips for garnishing

Directions:
1. Add all the listed ingredients to a blender
2. Blend until you have a smooth and creamy texture
3. Serve chilled and enjoy!

Nutrition Info: Calories: 132; Fat: 2.6g; Carbohydrates: 23.8g; Protein: 7.2g

WEIGHT LOSS SMOOTHIES

Leeks And Broccoli Cucumber Glass

Servings: 2
Cooking Time: 5 Minutes
Ingredients:
- 1 cup crushed ice
- 1 tablespoon Matcha
- ½ cup leaf lettuce, chopped
- ½ cup lettuce, chopped
- 1 lime, juiced
- 2 cucumbers, diced
- 2 leeks, chopped
- 2 tablespoons cashew butter
- 1 cup broccoli, diced

Directions:
1. Add all the ingredients except vegetables/fruits first
2. Blend until smooth
3. Add the vegetable/fruits
4. Blend until smooth
5. Add a few ice cubes and serve the smoothie
6. Enjoy!

Nutrition Info: Calories: 219; Fat: 6g; Carbohydrates: 6g; Protein: 4g

Spinach, Carrot And Tomato Smoothie

Servings: 2
Cooking Time: 2 Minutes
Ingredients:
- 1 cup fresh spinach, chopped
- 1-2 celery stalks chopped
- 1 small carrot, peeled and chopped
- 1 large tomato, chopped
- 1 small bell pepper, deseeded and chopped
- ¼ small onion
- 3-4 sprigs of cilantro leaves, chopped
- ½ sweet lime, Peeled and deseeded
- 1 ¼ cup of filtered water

Directions:
1. Place everything into the blender and run it on high for 30 seconds. Pour into serving glasses and enjoy.

Nutrition Info: (Per Serving): Calories- 74, Fat- 0.8 g, Protein- 3.5 g, Carbohydrates- 16.5 g

Chia-blueberry Smoothie

Servings: 2
Cooking Time: 5 Minutes
Ingredients:
- ½ cup blueberries, (fresh or frozen)
- 6 ounces of plain or Greek yogurt
- ½ banana, chopped
- 1 tablespoons Chia seeds, soaked
- A pinch of cinnamon powder
- 4 ounces of filtered water

Directions:
1. Add all the ingredients into the blender jar and pulse it on high for 30 seconds or until smooth.

Nutrition Info: (Per Serving): Calories- 325, Fat- 20 g, Protein-8 g, Carbohydrates-32 g

Healthy Raspberry And Coconut Glass

Servings: 1
Cooking Time: 10 Minutes
Ingredients:
- ¼ cup raspberries
- 1 tablespoon pepitas
- 1 tablespoon coconut oil
- ½ cup of coconut milk
- 1 cup 50/50 salad mix
- 1 ½ cups of water
- 1 pack stevia

Directions:
1. Add listed ingredients to a blender
2. Blend until you have a smooth and creamy texture
3. Serve chilled and enjoy!

Nutrition Info: Calories: 408; Fat: 41g; Carbohydrates: 10g; Protein: 5g

Banana And Spinach Raspberry Smoothie

Servings: 2
Cooking Time: 5 Minutes
Ingredients:
- 1 tablespoons cilantro
- 1 cup crushed ice
- 1 tablespoon ground flaxseed
- ½ cup raspberries
- 2 dates
- 2 bananas
- 1 cup spinach, chopped

Directions:
1. Add all the ingredients except vegetables/fruits first
2. Blend until smooth
3. Add the vegetable/fruits
4. Blend until smooth
5. Add a few ice cubes and serve the smoothie
6. Enjoy!

Nutrition Info: Calories: 120; Fat: 2g; Carbohydrates: 30g; Protein: 3g

Mint And Kale Smoothie

Servings: 2
Cooking Time: 5 Minutes
Ingredients:
- 1 cup kale, stems removed and chopped
- 6-7 fresh mint leaves, washed
- 1 green avocado, pitted, peeled and chopped
- 1 tablespoon chlorella powder
- 1 cup filtered water
- 3-4 ice cubes (optional)

Directions:
1. Add all the ingredients to the blender and process for 30 seconds on high.

Nutrition Info: (Per Serving): Calories- 280, Fat- 17.5 g, Protein- 19 g, Carbohydrates- 16 g

Flax And Almond Butter Smoothie

Servings: 2
Cooking Time: 5 Minutes
Ingredients:
- 1 teaspoon flaxseed
- ½ cup crushed ice
- 3 strawberries
- 1 banana, frozen
- 2 cups spinach
- 2 tablespoons almond butter
- ½ cup plain yogurt

Directions:
1. Add all the ingredients except vegetables/fruits first
2. Blend until smooth
3. Add the vegetable/fruits
4. Blend until smooth
5. Add a few ice cubes and serve the smoothie
6. Enjoy!

Nutrition Info: Calories: 147; Fat: 7g; Carbohydrates: 21g; Protein: 4g

Spiced Pineapple Smoothie

Servings: 2
Cooking Time: 5 Minutes
Ingredients:
- 1 cup pineapple, chopped (fresh or frozen)
- 1 large banana, chopped
- 2 tablespoons freshly squeezed lemon juice
- 1 teaspoon freshly grated ginger
- 1 tablespoon maca powder
- 1 tablespoon flax seed powder
- ¼ teaspoon cayenne pepper
- 1 ¼ cup filtered water

Directions:
1. Pour all the ingredients into the blender and process it for 45 seconds on medium speed and serve.

Nutrition Info: (Per Serving): Calories- 255, Fat- 3.8 g, Protein- 4.5 g, Carbohydrates- 57 g

Zucchini Apple Smoothie

Servings: 2
Cooking Time: 5 Minutes
Ingredients:
- 1½ cups crushed ice
- 1 tablespoon Spirulina
- 1 lemon, juiced
- 1 stalk celery
- ¾ avocado
- 2 apples, quartered
- ½ cup zucchini, diced

Directions:
1. Add all the ingredients except vegetables/fruits first
2. Blend until smooth
3. Add the vegetable/fruits
4. Blend until smooth
5. Add a few ice cubes and serve the smoothie
6. Enjoy!

Nutrition Info: Calories: 80; Fat: 4g; Carbohydrates: 11g; Protein: 2g

A-b-c Smoothie

Servings: 1-2
Cooking Time: 2 Minutes
Ingredients:
- 1 cup unsweetened almond milk
- 2 large bananas (fresh or frozen)
- 1 teaspoon Chia seeds, soaked
- 1 tablespoon almond butter
- 1 teaspoon vanilla extract
- 1 teaspoon pomegranate seeds for garnish

Directions:
1. To your blender, add all the items and process until you get a thick and creamy smoothie.
2. Pour into a glass and enjoy.

Nutrition Info: (Per Serving): Calories- 184, Fat- 6.6 g, Protein- 3.6 g, Carbohydrates- 30 g

Straight Up Avocado And Kale Smoothie

Servings: 2
Cooking Time: 5 Minutes
Ingredients:
- 1 tablespoon spirulina

- 1 cup chamomile tea
- 1 tablespoon Chia seeds
- 1 stalk celery
- 1 cup cucumber
- ½ avocado, diced
- 1 cup kale, chopped

Directions:
1. Add all the ingredients except vegetables/fruits first
2. Blend until smooth
3. Add the vegetable/fruits
4. Blend until smooth
5. Add a few ice cubes and serve the smoothie
6. Enjoy!

Nutrition Info: Calories: 236; Fat: 6g; Carbohydrates: 46g; Protein: 4g

Blueberry–avocado Smoothie

Servings: 1
Cooking Time: 2 Minutes
Ingredients:
- ½ cup blueberries (fresh or frozen)
- 3 tablespoons ripe avocado flesh
- 1 tablespoon Chia seeds, soaked for 10 minutes
- 1 teaspoon pure coconut oil
- ½ tablespoon raw organic honey
- A large pinch of cinnamon powder
- 1 cup filtered water

Directions:
1. Place all the above listed ingredients into your blender and pulse until smooth.

Nutrition Info: (Per Serving): Calories-330, Fat- 25 g, Protein- 4 g, Carbohydrates- 30 g

Raspberry- Grapefruit Smoothie

Servings: 2-3
Cooking Time: 5 Minutes
Ingredients:
- 2 cups fresh spinach, chopped
- ½ grapefruits, peeled and de seeded
- ½ cup raspberries (fresh or frozen)
- 1 California orange, peeled and de seeded
- ¼ cup whole strawberries (fresh or frozen)
- 1 tablespoon Chia seeds, soaked
- 1 ½ cups of filtered water

Directions:
1. To your blender, add all the items listed above and blend until smooth and creamy.

Nutrition Info: (Per Serving): Calories- 164, Fat- 5.5 g, Protein- 5.6 g, Carbohydrates- 29 g

Banana, Almond, And Dark Chocolate Smoothie

Servings: 2
Cooking Time: 5 Minutes
Ingredients:
- 1 cup banana, sliced
- 4 tablespoons dark chocolate, grated 80% cocoa
- 8 almonds, soaked overnight
- ½ cup milk, low-fat and chilled

Directions:
1. Toss the sliced bananas, grated dark chocolate, almonds, and chilled milk
2. Add all the listed ingredients to a blender
3. Blend until you have a smooth and creamy texture
4. Serve chilled and enjoy!

Nutrition Info: Calories: 114; Fat: 1g; Carbohydrates: 22g; Protein: 5g

Pumpkin Pie Buttered Coffee

Servings: 1
Cooking Time: 10 Minutes
Ingredients:
- 2 tablespoons pumpkin, canned
- 12 ounces hot coffee
- ¼ teaspoon pumpkin pie spice
- 1 tablespoon regular butter, unsalted
- Liquid stevia, to sweetened

Directions:
1. Add all the listed ingredients to a blender
2. Blend until you have a smooth and creamy texture
3. Serve chilled and enjoy!

Nutrition Info: Calories: 120; Fat: 12g; Carbohydrates: 2g; Protein: 1g

Banana-mango Delight

Servings: 2 Small
Cooking Time: 2 Minutes
Ingredients:
- ½ cup mango, chopped (fresh or frozen)
- ½ cup pineapple, chopped
- 1 large banana, chopped (fresh or frozen)
- ¾ cup plain or Greek yogurt
- 2 tablespoons flax seed powder
- 2-3 cubes of ice (optional)

Directions:
1. Add the fruits, ice, yogurt and yogurt into the blender and puree it until thick and creamy.

Nutrition Info: (Per Serving): Calories- 370, Fat- 7 g, Protein- 22 g, Carbohydrates-61 g

Coconutty Apple Smoothie

Servings: 1
Cooking Time: 2 Minutes
Ingredients:
- 1 cup apple, cored and chopped
- ½ cup organic coconut milk
- 1 small banana, chopped
- 2 teaspoons almond butter
- ½ cup kale, chopped
- 1 ½ teaspoon flaxseed powder
- ½ teaspoon cinnamon powder

Directions:
1. Combine all the ingredients together in the blender and pulse for 30 seconds. Pour into a glass and enjoy.

Nutrition Info: (Per Serving): Calories- 330, Fat- 14 g, Protein- 5.8 g, Carbohydrates- 51 g

Flax And Kiwi Spinach Smoothie

Servings: 2
Cooking Time: 5 Minutes
Ingredients:
- 1 cup crushed ice
- 3 tablespoons ground flax
- 3 kiwis, diced
- 1 stalk celery, chopped
- 1 banana, chopped
- 2 apples, quartered
- 1 cup spinach, chopped

Directions:
1. Add all the ingredients except vegetables/fruits first
2. Blend until smooth
3. Add the vegetable/fruits
4. Blend until smooth
5. Add a few ice cubes and serve the smoothie
6. Enjoy!

Nutrition Info: Calories: 142; Fat: 7g; Carbohydrates: 16g; Protein: 6g

Clemintine Dreamsicle Smoothie

Servings: 1
Cooking Time: 2 Minutes
Ingredients:
- 4 Clementine, peeled and chopped
- 1 small banana (fresh or frozen)
- ¼ cup unsweetened almond milk
- ½ teaspoon raw organic honey
- ½ teaspoon vanilla extract
- A pinch of turmeric powder
- A pinch of Celtic salt
- 3-4 ice cubes

Directions:
1. Place the ingredients listed above into your high speed blender and process until the smoothie is thick and creamy.

Nutrition Info: (Per Serving): Calories- 145, Fat- 0.3 g, Protein- 6.6 g, Carbohydrates- 33.5 g

Cucumber Kale And Lime Apple Smoothie

Servings: 2
Cooking Time: 5 Minutes
Ingredients:
- 1 cup crushed ice
- 1 cucumber, diced
- ¼ cup raspberries, chopped
- 1 lime, juiced
- 1 avocado, diced
- 2 apples, quartered
- 1 cup kale, chopped

Directions:
1. Add all the ingredients except vegetables/fruits first
2. Blend until smooth
3. Add the vegetable/fruits
4. Blend until smooth
5. Add a few ice cubes and serve the smoothie
6. Enjoy!

Nutrition Info: Calories: 291; Fat: 2g; Carbohydrates: 38g; Protein: 7g

Peanut Butter, Banana And Cacao Smoothie

Servings: 2
Cooking Time: 5 Minutes
Ingredients:
- 1 cup unsweetened almond milk
- 2 tablespoons peanut butter
- 2 large ripe bananas (fresh or frozen)
- 2 teaspoons cacao powder
- ½ teaspoon vanilla extract
- 1 teaspoon raw organic honey
- 3-4 cubes of ice

Directions:
1. Add all the ingredients in the blender and process until smooth.

Nutrition Info: (Per Serving): Calories- 345, Fat- 16 g, Protein- 11 g, Carbohydrates- 90 g

Meanie-greenie Weigh Loss Smoothie

Servings: 2-3
Cooking Time: 5 Minutes

Ingredients:
- 1 cup kale, stems removed
- 1 cup green cucumber, de-seeded and chopped
- 1 celery stalk, chopped
- 1 small pear, peeled, cored and chopped
- 1 teaspoon freshly grated ginger
- A handful of parsley
- 1 ½ cups of filtered water
- 1 teaspoon freshly squeezed lemon juice

Directions:
1. Place all the ingredients in the order listed above and pulse until the desired consistency is attained.

Nutrition Info: (Per Serving): Calories- 64.3, Fat- 0.3 g, Protein- 1 g, Carbohydrates- 15.8 g

Grape And Spinach Smoothie

Servings: 2
Cooking Time: 5 Minutes
Ingredients:
- 2 cups fresh spinach, chopped
- 1 large pear, peeled, cored and chopped
- 1 cup grapes, washed (red or green)
- 2 tablespoons avocado flesh
- 3 teaspoons freshly squeezed lime juice
- ¾ cup plain or Greek yogurt

Directions:
1. Whizz up all the ingredients in the blender for 45 seconds and serve.

Nutrition Info: (Per Serving): Calories- 315, Fat-6 g, Protein- 21 g, Carbohydrates-52 g

Carrot Spice Smoothie

Servings: 2
Cooking Time: 5 Minutes
Ingredients:
- 1 cup unsweetened almond milk
- 1 ripe banana, chopped
- 1 cup carrots, peeled and chopped
- 4 ounces plain yogurt
- 1 tablespoon raw organic honey
- ¼ teaspoon freshly grated ginger
- ¼ teaspoon cinnamon powder
- A pinch of nutmeg powder
- 3-4 ice cubes

Directions:
1. Add all the ingredients into the blender one by one and pulse until thick and creamy.

Nutrition Info: (Per Serving): Calories- 295, Fat- 3.5 g, Protein- 9 g, Carbohydrates- 61.5 g

Veggie Wonder

Servings: 2
Cooking Time: 2 Minutes
Ingredients:
- 1 cup fresh spinach, washed and chopped
- 1 largest carrot, peeled and chopped
- 1 celery stalk, chopped
- 1/3 cup red beet, peeled and chopped
- 3-4 sprigs of parsley
- 1 large tomato, chopped
- 1 ½ cups filtered water

Directions:
1. Combine the above listed ingredients in the blender and run it on medium high speed for 30 – 45 seconds.
2. Pour into tall glasses and serve.

Nutrition Info: (Per Serving): Calories- 76, Fat- 0.7 g, Protein- 3.5 g, Carbohydrates- 16.4 g

Berry-banana-spinach Smoothie

Servings: 2
Cooking Time: 5 Minutes
Ingredients:
- 1 cup mixed berries (fresh or frozen)
- 1 cup baby spinach, washed and chopped
- ½ large banana, chopped (fresh r frozen)
- 1 teaspoon coconut oil
- 1 tablespoon flax seeds
- ¼ teaspoon cayenne pepper powder
- 1 cup filtered water

Directions:
1. Place all the ingredients in the blender and run I on high for 30 seconds or until the desired consistency is got.

Nutrition Info: (Per Serving): Calories- 250, Fat-14 g, Protein-3 g, Carbohydrates-33 g

Mango Strawberry Smoothie

Servings: 1
Cooking Time: 10 Minutes
Ingredients:
- 1 cup Greek yogurt
- 2 mangoes, peeled, pit removed and chopped
- 4 teaspoons honey
- 3 cups strawberries, fresh or frozen
- 16 ice cubes

Directions:
1. Add all the listed ingredients to a blender
2. Blend until you have a smooth and creamy texture
3. Serve chilled and enjoy!

Nutrition Info: Calories: 394; Fat: 3.3g; Carbohydrates: 85.4g; Protein: 12.8g

Cherry-vanilla Smoothie

Servings: 1
Cooking Time: 5 Minutes
Ingredients:
- 1/3 cup unsweetened almond milk
- ½ cup plain yogurt
- ¼ cup rolled oats
- 1 cup cherries (fresh or frozen)
- 1 teaspoon raw organic honey
- ½ teaspoon almond flakes
- ½ teaspoon vanilla extract

Directions:
1. Load your blender with all the above listed ingredients and blend on medium speed for 20 -30 seconds till a creamy mixture is got.

Nutrition Info: (Per Serving): Calories- 115, Fat- 1.8 g, Protein- 5.0 g, Carbohydrates- 20 g

Green Tea- Mango Smoothie

Servings: 2
Cooking Time: 10 Minutes
Ingredients:
- 1 cup mango, chopped (fresh or frozen)
- 1 cup green tea
- 1 cup fresh spinach, chopped
- ½ cup avocado, chopped
- 1 teaspoon coconut oil
- ½ teaspoon raw organic honey
- A inch of Celtic salt

Directions:
1. First, prepare a cup of your favorite green tea and allow w it to cool to room temperature.
2. Once the tea has cooled, combine all the ingredients in the high speed blender and whizz until thick and creamy.
3. Serve and enjoy!

Nutrition Info: (Per Serving): Calories-330, Fat- 21 g, Protein- 4g, Carbohydrates- 35 g

Kale Celery Smoothie

Servings: 2
Cooking Time: 10 Minutes
Ingredients:
- 3 cups kale, chopped
- 2 stalks celery, diced
- 1 red apple, cored and diced
- 2 cups almond milk, unsweetened
- 1 ¼ cups ice
- 2 teaspoons honey
- 2 tablespoons flaxseed, ground

Directions:
1. Add all the listed ingredients to a blender
2. Blend until you have a smooth and creamy texture
3. Serve chilled and enjoy!

Nutrition Info: Calories: 341; Fat: 29.8g; Carbohydrates: 18.6g; Protein: 5.3g

KID FRIENDLY HEALTHY SMOOTHIES

Banana-cado Smoothie

Servings: 3
Cooking Time: 5 Minutes
Ingredients:
- 1 cup fresh organic coconut water
- ½ cup unsweetened almond milk
- ½ cup unsweetened coconut milk
- 1 ripe banana, chopped
- 2 teaspoons chia sees
- 2 tablespoons fresh avocado flesh

Directions:
1. Place all the above ingredients into the blender jar and process until the mixture is thick and creamy.

Nutrition Info: (Per Serving): Calories- 465, Fat- 7 g, Protein- 7 g, Carbohydrates- 13 g

Mixed Fruit Madness

Servings: 1
Cooking Time: 10 Minutes
Ingredients:
- 1 cup spring mix salad blend
- 2 cups water
- 3 medium blackberries, whole
- 1 packet Stevia, optional
- 1 tablespoon avocado oil
- 1 tablespoon coconut flakes shredded and unsweetened
- 2 tablespoons pecans, chopped
- 1 tablespoon hemp seeds
- 1 tablespoon sunflower seeds

Directions:
1. Add all the ingredients except vegetables/fruits first
2. Blend until smooth
3. Add the vegetable/fruits
4. Blend until smooth
5. Add a few ice cubes and serve the smoothie
6. Enjoy!

Nutrition Info: Calories: 150; Fat: 2g; Carbohydrates: 37g; Protein: 3g

Date Pomegranate Wonder

Servings: 3
Cooking Time: 5 Minutes
Ingredients:
- 1 cup whole blueberries (fresh or frozen)
- 1 cup unsweetened, fresh coconut milk
- ½ cup baby spinach, washed and chopped
- ½ cup pomegranate seeds
- 5-6 dates, pitted
- 2 teaspoons Chia seeds, soaked
- 4-5 ice cubes (optional)

Directions:
1. Whizz up all the ingredients in a blender, pour into glass and serve!

Nutrition Info: (Per Serving): Calories- 525, Fat- 18 g, Protein- 7 g, Carbohydrates- 100 g

Apple Berry Smoothie

Servings: 2
Cooking Time: 10 Minutes
Ingredients:
- 2 large apples
- 4 cups spinach
- 2 cups berries, mixed
- 2 cups of water

Directions:
1. Add all the listed ingredients to a blender
2. Blend until you have a smooth and creamy texture
3. Serve chilled and enjoy!

Nutrition Info: Calories: 210; Fat: 1.1g; Carbohydrates: 50g; Protein: 3.3g

Pineapple Banana Smoothie

Servings: 2
Cooking Time: 10 Minutes
Ingredients:
- 2 apples
- 4 cups spinach
- 2 bananas
- 2 cups pineapples
- 2 cups of water

Directions:
1. Add all the listed ingredients to a blender
2. Blend until you have a smooth and creamy texture
3. Serve chilled and enjoy!

Nutrition Info: Calories: 317; Fat: 1.2g; Carbohydrates: 81.6g; Protein: 4.5g

Peanut Butter Broccoli Smoothie

Servings: 3
Cooking Time: 5 Minutes
Ingredients:
- 1 cup unsweetened almond milk
- 1 cup fresh spinach, washed and chopped
- 1 cup broccoli florets, washed and chopped
- 1 large kale leaf, washed and chopped

- 1 ripe banana, chopped
- 2 teaspoons peanut butter
- 1 teaspoon raw organic honey (optional)

Directions:
1. Add all the ingredients into the high speed blender and whizz until smooth.

Nutrition Info: (Per Serving): Calories- 325, Fat- 14 g, Protein- 10 g, Carbohydrates- 46 g

Berry Peachy Blush

Servings: 3
Cooking Time: 2 Minutes
Ingredients:
- 1 cup fresh, unsweetened coconut milk
- 1 cup whole strawberries (fresh or frozen)
- ¾ cup peaches, pitted (fresh or frozen)
- A small ripe banana, chopped
- 3 teaspoons raw organic honey
- ¼ cup filtered water
- 4-5 ice cubes

Directions:
1. Place all the above ingredients into the blender jar and process until the mixture is thick and creamy.

Nutrition Info: (Per Serving): Calories- 385, Fat- 20 g, Protein- 4.2 g, Carbohydrates- 51 g

The Overloaded Berry Shake

Servings: 1
Cooking Time: 10 Minutes
Ingredients:
- ½ cup whole milk yogurt
- 1 pack stevia
- ¼ cup raspberries
- ¼ cup blackberry
- ¼ cup strawberries, chopped
- 1 tablespoon cocoa powder
- 1 tablespoon avocado oil
- 1½ cups water

Directions:
1. Add all the ingredients except vegetables/fruits first
2. Blend until smooth
3. Add the vegetable/fruits
4. Blend until smooth
5. Add a few ice cubes and serve the smoothie
6. Enjoy!

Nutrition Info: Calories: 200; Fat: 7g; Carbohydrates: 24g; Protein: 2g

Kale, Cucumber Cooler

Servings: 2
Cooking Time: 2 Minutes
Ingredients:
- 1 large cup whole strawberries (fresh or frozen)
- 1 cup pineapple, peeled and chopped
- ½ cup green cucumber, chopped
- 2-3 large kale leaves, chopped
- 2 teaspoons freshly squeezed lemon juice
- ½ teaspoon raw organic honey
- 2-3 ice cubes

Directions:
1. Add all the above ingredients into your blender jar and pulse until thick and frothy

Nutrition Info: (Per Serving): Calories- 152, Fat- 0.6 g, Protein- 3.8 g, Carbohydrates- 35 g

Pineapple Papaya Perfection Smoothie

Servings: 3
Cooking Time: 5 Minutes
Ingredients:
- 2 cups papaya. Peeled and chopped
- 1 cup plain low fat yogurt
- ½ cup pineapple, peeled and chopped
- 1 teaspoon grated coconut
- 1 teaspoon flax seed powder
- 2 teaspoon freshly squeezed lemon juice
- 4-5 ice cubes

Directions:
1. To make this smoothie, place everything into the blender and pulse until smooth. Serve immediately.

Nutrition Info: (Per Serving): Calories- 230, Fat- 1.4 g, Protein- 12.5 g, Carbohydrates- 65 g

Chilled Watermelon Krush

Servings: 2
Cooking Time: 2 Minutes
Ingredients:
- 2 cups watermelon, chopped (seedless)
- 5-6 fresh mint leaves, roughly torn
- ½ cup low fat, plain yogurt
- 1 ½ teaspoons raw organic honey
- 3-4 ice cubes

Directions:
1. Add all the above ingredients into your blender jar and pulse until thick and frothy.

Nutrition Info: (Per Serving): Calories- 185, Fat- 0 g, Protein- 13 g, Carbohydrates- 35 g

Mesmerizing Strawberry And Chocolate Shake

Servings: 1
Cooking Time: 10 Minutes
Ingredients:
- ½ cup heavy cream, liquid
- 1 tablespoon cocoa powder
- 1 pack stevia
- ½ cup strawberry, sliced
- 1 tablespoon coconut flakes, unsweetened
- 1½ cups water

Directions:
1. Add all the ingredients except vegetables/fruits first
2. Blend until smooth
3. Add the vegetable/fruits
4. Blend until smooth
5. Add a few ice cubes and serve the smoothie
6. Enjoy!

Nutrition Info: Calories: 453; Fat: 22g; Carbohydrates: 39g; Protein: 10g

Very Berry Blueberry Wonder

Servings: 2
Cooking Time: 5 Minutes
Ingredients:
- ½ cup whole blueberries (fresh or frozen)
- 1 tangerine, peeled and seeded
- 1 medium beet, peeled and chopped
- ½ large banana, chopped (fresh or frozen)
- 1 tablespoons chia seed
- A large pinch of cinnamon powder
- 1/3 cup low fat plain yogurt
- 4-5 ice cubes

Directions:
1. Whizz up all the ingredients in a blender, pour into glass and serve!

Nutrition Info: (Per Serving): Calories-285, Fat- 4 g, Protein- 20 g, Carbohydrates- 50 g

Raw Chocolate Smoothie

Servings: 2
Cooking Time: 10 Minutes
Ingredients:
- 2 medium bananas
- 4 tablespoons peanut butter, raw
- 1 cup almond milk
- 3 tablespoons cocoa powder, raw
- 2 tablespoons honey, raw

Directions:
1. Add all the listed ingredients to a blender

2. Blend until you have a smooth and creamy texture
3. Serve chilled and enjoy!

Nutrition Info: Calories: 217; Fat: 2.8g; Carbohydrates: 52.7g; Protein: 3.4g

Ultimate Berry Blush

Servings: 4
Cooking Time: 5 Minutes
Ingredients:
- 2 cups mixed berries (fresh or frozen)
- 2 cups low fat plain yogurt
- 2 large bananas, chopped (fresh r frozen0
- 1 teaspoon cashews
- 4-5 ice cubes

Directions:
1. Combine all the ingredients in a high speed blender and whirr until thick and smooth.

Nutrition Info: (Per Serving): Calories- 150, Fat- 1.5 g, Protein- 5 g, Carbohydrates- 30 g

Delish Pineapple And Coconut Milk Smoothie

Servings: 2
Cooking Time: 5 Minutes
Ingredients:
- ¾ cup of coconut water
- ¼ cup pineapple, frozen

Directions:
1. Add listed ingredients to a blender
2. Blend on high until you have a smooth and creamy texture
3. Serve chilled and enjoy!

Nutrition Info: Calories: 132; Fat: 12g; Carbohydrates: 7g; Protein: 1g

Cool Coco-loco Cream Shake

Servings: 1
Cooking Time: 10 Minutes
Ingredients:
- ½ cup coconut milk
- 2 tablespoons Dutch-processed cocoa powder, unsweetened
- 1 cup brewed coffee, chilled
- 1-2 packs stevia
- 1 tablespoon hemp seeds

Directions:
1. Add all the ingredients except vegetables/fruits first
2. Blend until smooth
3. Add the vegetable/fruits

4. Blend until smooth
5. Add a few ice cubes and serve the smoothie
6. Enjoy!

Nutrition Info: Calories: 337; Fat: 11g; Carbohydrates: 38g; Protein: 1g

Directions:
1. Place all the ingredients into the blender and puree until everything is well combined.

Nutrition Info: (Per Serving): Calories- 400, Fat- 3 g, Protein- 4 g, Carbohydrates- 10 g

Carrot Peach Blush

Servings: 2-3
Cooking Time: 5 Minutes
Ingredients:
- 1 cup unsweetened almond milk
- 1 ripe banana, chopped
- 2 large peaches, pitted and chopped
- 1 large carrot, peeled and chopped
- 1 teaspoon freshly grated ginger
- 3-4 ice cubes

Directions:
1. To your high speed blender, add all the above mentioned items and process on high for 30 seconds. Pour into serving glasses and enjoy immediately.

Nutrition Info: (Per Serving): Calories- 110, Fat- 5 g, Protein- 2 g, Carbohydrates- 15 g

Blueberry Pineapple Blast Smoothie

Servings: 2
Cooking Time: 2 Minutes
Ingredients:
- 1 cup freshly squeezed pineapple juice
- 1/3 cup fresh, organic coconut milk
- 1 cup whole blueberries (fresh or frozen)
- 2 teaspoons of shredded coconut
- 3-4 ice cubes

Directions:
1. Add all the ingredients into the blender jar and pulse it on high for 30 seconds or until smooth.

Nutrition Info: (Per Serving): Calories- 265, Fat- 10 g, Protein- 3 g, Carbohydrates- 45 g

Chocolate Spinach Smoothie

Servings: 4
Cooking Time: 10 Minutes
Ingredients:
- 4 cups banana, sliced
- 2 cups spinach, packed
- 6 tablespoons peanut butter
- 2 cups almond milk
- ½ cup of cocoa powder
- 2 tablespoons flaxseeds, grounded

Directions:
1. Add all the listed ingredients to a blender
2. Blend until you have a smooth and creamy texture
3. Serve chilled and enjoy!

Nutrition Info: Calories: 356; Fat: 16.2g; Carbohydrates: 51.7g; Protein: 13g

Cocoa Banana Smoothie

Servings: 4
Cooking Time: 10 Minutes
Ingredients:
- 4 large bananas, peeled and sliced
- ½ cup creamy peanut butter
- 2 cups almond milk
- 4 tablespoons cocoa powder, unsweetened
- 1 teaspoon vanilla extract
- 2 cups ice

Directions:
1. Add all the listed ingredients to a blender
2. Blend until you have a smooth and creamy texture
3. Serve chilled and enjoy!

Nutrition Info: Calories: 346; Fat: 17.4g; Carbohydrates: 46.1g; Protein: 10g

Coconut Strawberry Punch

Servings: 2
Cooking Time: 5 Minutes
Ingredients:
- 1 cup fresh coconut water
- 8 – 10 whole strawberries (fresh or frozen)
- ½ cup plain yogurt
- 1 tablespoon freshly squeezed lemon juice
- 2-3 ice cubes

Raspberry Pecan Date Delight

Servings: 1 Large
Cooking Time: 2 Minutes
Ingredients:
- 1 ripe banana, chopped
- ½ cup whole raspberries (fresh or frozen)
- 1 teaspoon coconut oil
- 1 tablespoon pecan halves
- 1 date, pitted
- 1 teaspoon flaxseed powder
- 1 cup filtered water

Directions:
1. Pour all the ingredients into your blender and process until smooth.
Nutrition Info: (Per Serving): Calories- 375, Fat- 15 g, Protein- 3.5 g, Carbohydrates- 65 g

Delicious Creamy Choco Shake

Servings: 1
Cooking Time: 10 Minutes
Ingredients:
- ½ cup heavy cream
- 2 tablespoons cocoa powder
- 1 pack stevia
- 1 cup water

Directions:
1. Add all the ingredients except vegetables/fruits first
2. Blend until smooth
3. Add the vegetable/fruits
4. Blend until smooth
5. Add a few ice cubes and serve the smoothie
6. Enjoy!

Nutrition Info: Calories: 180; Fat: 6g; Carbohydrates: 30g; Protein: 3g

Beet Berry Chiller

Servings: 2
Cooking Time: 2 Minutes
Ingredients:
- ¾ cup freshly prepared cranberry juice (unsweetened)
- A small handful of cranberries (fresh or frozen)
- 1 cup raw beet, peeled and chopped
- 4-5 whole strawberries (fresh or frozen)
- 1 tablespoon raw organic honey
- 2 teaspoons freshly squeezed lemon juice
- 4- ice cubes

Directions:
1. Pour all the ingredients into your blender jar and process until smooth.
Nutrition Info: (Per Serving): Calories- 90, Fat- 0 g, Protein- 1.2 g, Carbohydrates- 22 g

Peanut Butter Jelly Smoothie

Servings: 2
Cooking Time: 2 Minutes
Ingredients:
- 1 cup whole raspberries (fresh or frozen)
- 2 teaspoons peanut butter
- ½ large banana, chopped
- 1 cup unsweetened almond milk
- ½ teaspoon raw organic honey
- 2-3 ice cubes

Directions:
1. Pour all the ingredients into your blender and process until smooth.
Nutrition Info: (Per Serving): Calories-270, Fat- 12 g, Protein- 7 g, Carbohydrates- 40 g

HEART HEALTHY SMOOTHIES

Almond- Citrus Punch

Servings: 2
Cooking Time: 2 Minutes
Ingredients:
- 1 cup unsweetened almond milk
- ½ cup freshly squeezed orange juice
- 1 tablespoon raw organic honey
- 1/3 cup freshly squeezed lime juice
- 1 tablespoon freshly squeezed lemon
- ¼ teaspoon vanilla extract
- A handful of ice cubes

Directions:
1. Pour all the ingredients into the blender and blend for 45 seconds until well combined.

Nutrition Info: (Per Serving): Calories- 150, Fat- 4 g, Protein- 2 g, Carbohydrates- 30 g

Ginger Banana Kick

Servings: 2
Cooking Time: 5 Minutes
Ingredients:
- 1 large banana, chopped (fresh or frozen)
- 1 large orange, peeled and de seeded
- 2 cups almond milk or plain soy milk
- 1 teaspoon freshly grated ginger
- ¼ teaspoon vanilla extract
- ½ teaspoon raw, organic honey (optional)
- 1 few ice cubes

Directions:
1. Load your blender jar with the ingredients listed above and puree it until nice and thick.

Nutrition Info: (Per Serving): Calories- 181, Fat- 5.1 g, Proteins- 8.3 g, Carbohydrates- 30 g

Berry Banana Smoothie

Servings: 1
Cooking Time: 5 Minutes
Ingredients:
- 1 large orange, peeled and chopped
- 2 cups of mixed greens or baby spinach, washed
- 1 cup mixed berries (fresh or frozen)
- 1 banana, peeled and chopped
- 1-2 tablespoons avocado flesh
- 1 tablespoon of flax seeds, powdered
- 1 cup filtered water

Directions:
1. First add the liquids and the fruits to your blender, next add the greens and flax seeds and sauce the lid.
2. Process for 30 seconds on high or until the smoothie is thick and creamy.

Nutrition Info: (Per Serving): Calories- 334, Fat-8 g, Protein- 6 g, Carbohydrates- 65 g

Lime And Melon Healer

Servings: 1 Large
Cooking Time: 2 Minutes
Ingredients:
- 1 cup cantaloupe, peeled, deseeded and chopped
- 1 cup honeydew melon, peeled, deseeded and chopped
- Freshly squeezed juice of 1 lime
- 2 teaspoons of raw organic honey
- A pinch of cayenne pepper
- 2-3 cubes of ice (optional)

Directions:
1. Whizz up all the ingredients in your blender, pour into a glass and enjoy!

Nutrition Info: (Per Serving): Calories- 98, Fat- 0 g, Protein-0 g, Carbohydrates- 14 g

Almond- Melon Punch

Servings: 2
Cooking Time: 2 Minutes
Ingredients:
- 2 cups watermelon, deseeded and chopped
- 2 teaspoon almonds, soaked and chopped
- ½ cup plain yogurt
- ½ teaspoon freshly grated ginger
- 1 teaspoon raw organic honey or liquid Stevia
- 3-4 ice cubes

Directions:
1. Add all the ingredients into the blender and pulse until well combined.

Nutrition Info: (Per Serving): Calories- 197, Fat- 2 g, Protein- 7 g, Carbohydrates- 45 g

Chia-cacao Melon Smoothie

Servings: 2
Cooking Time: 5 Minutes
Ingredients:
- 1 cup fresh strawberries
- 1 cup cantaloupe, chopped
- 1 large banana (fresh or frozen)
- 2 large chard leaves, chopped
- 1 cup unsweetened almond milk
- 1 tablespoon cacao powder
- 1 tablespoons Chia seeds, soaked

Directions:
1. Pour all the ingredients into your blender and whizz it up on high speed for 45 seconds or until done.
Nutrition Info: (Per Serving): Calories- 330, Fat- 0 g, Protein- 11 g, Carbohydrates- 62 g

Cinn-apple Beet Smoothie

Servings: 1
Cooking Time: 2 Minutes
Ingredients:
- 1 large red beet, peeled and chopped
- 1 large carrot, peeled and chopped
- 1 red apple, cored and chopped
- 1 teaspoon freshly grated ginger
- 1 teaspoon cinnamon powder
- 1 teaspoon coconut oil
- ½ cup filtered water
- ½ teaspoon raw organic honey

Directions:
1. Load your blender with all the ingredients and process it on medium for 30 seconds and then on high speed for 45 seconds or until well combined.
Nutrition Info: (Per Serving): Calories- 211, Fat- 6 g, Protein- 11 g, Carbohydrates- 44 g

Almond-banana Blend

Servings: 3
Cooking Time: 5 Minutes
Ingredients:
- 4 large, ripe bananas (fresh or frozen)
- 1 cup unsweetened almond milk
- 2 tablespoons almonds (soaked and chopped)
- 1 cup plain yogurt
- 3 teaspoons raw organic honey

Directions:
1. Pour all the ingredients into the blender and puree until a creamy smoothie is got.
Nutrition Info: (Per Serving): Calories- 192, Fat- 5 g, Protein- 5 g, Carbohydrates- 38 g

Spinach And Grape Smoothie

Servings: 1 Large
Cooking Time: 5 Minutes
Ingredients:
- 1 cup red grapes (seedless)
- 2 cups baby spinach
- 1 banana (fresh or frozen)
- 1 tablespoon Chia seeds (soaked)
- 1 teaspoon freshly squeezed lemon juice
- A handful of ice cubes

Directions:
1. Load all the ingredients into your blender jar and secure it tightly with a lid.
2. Pulse it on medium speed for 30 seconds and on high for 1 minute or until smooth.
Nutrition Info: (Per Serving): Calories-107, Fat-2.4 g, Protein-1.5 g, Carbohydrates-26.5 g

Mint And Avocado Smoothie

Servings: 3
Cooking Time: 5 Minutes
Ingredients:
- 2 cups unsweetened almond milk
- 1 medium banana, chopped
- 2 cups of fresh spinach
- 1 kiwi, peeled and quartered
- Freshly squeezed juice of 1 lime
- 6-8 fresh mint leaves
- ½ avocado, pitted and chopped
- 1 teaspoon freshly grated ginger

Directions:
1. Place all the above listed ingredients in the same order into your blender jar and process it until thick and smooth.
Nutrition Info: (Per Serving): Calories- 254, Fat- 12 g, Protein-10 g, Carbohydrates- 31 g

Peach-ban-illa Smoothie

Servings: 2 Small
Cooking Time: 5 Minutes
Ingredients:
- 1 ¼ cup peaches, pitted and chopped
- 1 large banana (fresh or frozen)
- 1 cup plain yogurt
- 1 teaspoon vanilla extract
- 1 teaspoon Chia seeds, soaked
- A handful of ice

Directions:
1. Combine all the ingredients in the blender and blend until the desired consistency is got.
Nutrition Info: (Per Serving): Calories- 170, Fat- 2 g, Protein- 5 g, Carbohydrates- 45 g

Melon And Soy Smoothie

Servings: 2
Cooking Time: 5 Minutes
Ingredients:
- 1 green cucumber, chopped
- 2 cups melon, chopped

- 1 ½ cups soybeans, boiled
- 4-5 fresh basil leaves
- 4-5 ice cubes

Directions:
1. Add all the ingredients into the blender and process it for 1 minute or until done.

Nutrition Info: (Per Serving): Calories- 200, Fat- 1.5 g, Protein- 10 g, Carbohydtaets-48 g

Mango-ginger Tango

Servings: 2
Cooking Time: 5 Minutes
Ingredients:
- 1 cup pineapple, peeled and chopped
- 1 cup mango, chopped
- 1 large orange, peeled and de seeded
- ½ cup filtered water
- 2 cups fresh kale, stems removed and chopped
- 1 teaspoon freshly grated ginger
- 2-3 cubes of ice

Directions:
1. Place all the ingredients into the blended one by one and pulse until smooth.

Nutrition Info: (Per Serving): Calories- 355, Fat- 0 g, Protein- 9 g, Carbohydrates- 88 g

Pineapple-pear And Spinach Smoothie

Servings: 2
Cooking Time: 5 Minutes
Ingredients:
- 1 cup pineapple, peeled and chopped
- ½ green pear, cored and chopped
- ¾ cup unsweetened almond milk
- 2 cups baby spinach
- 1 cup fresh kale
- 2 tablespoons Chia seeds, soaked
- ¼ teaspoon freshly grated ginger
- 1 teaspoon freshly squeezed lemon juice

Directions:
1. First add the fruits to your blender and whizz for 30 seconds until pureed.
2. Then add the rest f the ingredients and pulse for 1 minute or until a creamy smoothie is got.
3. Pour into tall glasses and enjoy!

Nutrition Info: (Per Serving): Caloris-340, Fat- 0 g, Protein- 8 g, Carbohydrates- 47 g

Oatmeal Banana Smoothie

Servings: 2 Small
Cooking Time: 5 Minutes
Ingredients:
- 1 large banana (fresh or frozen)
- 1 persimmon, peeled and chopped
- 1 cup mango, chopped (fresh or frozen)
- 4 tablespoons rolled oats, soaked
- 1 tablespoon raw organic honey
- A pinch of cinnamon powder

Directions:
1. Place all the ingredients into the blender and blend until creamy.

Nutrition Info: (Per Serving): Calories- 420, Fat- 2 g, Protein- 9 g, Carbohydrates- 95 g

Peach And Celery Smoothie

Servings: 2
Cooking Time: 5 Minutes
Ingredients:
- ½ green cucumber, chopped with peel on
- 1 large peach, pitted and chopped
- 1 orange, peeled and de seeded
- 2 tablespoons avocado flesh
- 2-3 stalks celery, washed and chopped
- 2 cups fresh Swiss chard, chopped
- ¾ cup filtered water
- 3-4 cubes of ice

Directions:
1. Combine all the above ingredients in your blender and process until the desired consistency is obtained.

Nutrition Info: (Per Serving): Calories- 255, Fat- 0 g, Protein- 8 g, Carbohydrates- 50 g

Vanilla- Mango Madness

Servings: 1
Cooking Time: 2 Minutes
Ingredients:
- 1 cup mango, chopped (fresh or frozen)
- 1 cup plain yogurt
- 1 tablespoon freshly squeezed lemon juice
- ¼ teaspoon vanilla extract
- ¼ teaspoon nutmeg powder
- 1 teaspoon raw organic honey
- A pinch of Celtic salt
- ¼ cup filtered water

Directions:
1. To your blender jar, add all the ingredients and whizz until thick and creamy.

Nutrition Info: (Per Serving): Calories- 160, Fat- 2 g, Protein- 7 g, Carbohydrates- 29.3 g

Hemp-avocado Smoothie

Servings: 2
Cooking Time: 5 Minutes
Ingredients:
- A red apple, cored and chopped
- 1 tablespoon avocado flesh
- 1 cup unsweetened almond milk
- 2 tablespoon hemp seeds
- 2 cups fresh baby spinach

Directions:
1. Pour all the ingredients into your blender and run in on high for 1 minute. Pour into tall glasses and enjoy!

Nutrition Info: (Per Serving): Calories- 350, Fat- 0 g, Protein- 10 g, Carbohydrates- 43 g

Beet And Apple Smoothie

Servings: 2
Cooking Time: 5 Minutes
Ingredients:
- 2 beetroots, peeled and chopped
- ½ cup blueberries, fresh or frozen
- 1 apple, cored, peeled and chipped
- 1 teaspoon freshly grated ginger
- 1 cup filtered water

Directions:
1. Combine all the ingredients in the blender and pulse it on high for 1 minute or until smooth.

Nutrition Info: (Per Serving): Calories-88, Fat- 0 g, Protein- 2 g, Carbohydrates- 20 g

Pina Berry Smoothie

Servings: 2
Cooking Time: 2 Minutes
Ingredients:
- 1 cup whole strawberries (fresh or frozen)
- 1 cup pineapple, chopped fresh or frozen)
- 1 teaspoon vanilla extract
- 1 cup plain yogurt
- 4-5 ice cubes

Directions:
1. Pour everything into the blender and blend until thick and frothy.

Nutrition Info: (Per Serving): Calories: 12, Fat-0.5 g, Protein-6 g, Carbohydrates-25 g

Oats And Berry Smoothie

Servings: 1
Cooking Time: 2 Minutes
Ingredients:
- 1 small ripe banana (fresh or frozen)
- 1 cup whole strawberries (fresh or frozen)
- ¼ cup almonds (soaked and de-skinned)
- ½ cup rolled oats
- 1 teaspoon raw organic honey
- 1/3 cup plain yogurt
- ¼ teaspoon vanilla extract

Directions:
1. Load the blender jar with all the above listed ingredients and process it for a minute until thick and creamy.
2. Pour into a glass and serve immediately!

Nutrition Info: (Per Serving): Calories- 450, Fat- 15.7 g, Protein- 17.5 g, Carbohydrates- 74 g

Kiwi-berry-nana

Servings: 2
Cooking Time: 5 Minutes
Ingredients:
- 1 cup whole strawberries (fresh or frozen)
- ½ cup blueberries (fresh or frozen)
- ¼ cup plain yogurt
- ½ cup fresh spinach
- ½ cup fresh kale, stems removed
- 1 kiwi, peeled and chopped
- 1 large banana (fresh or frozen)
- 1 cup filtered water
- 1 tablespoon pure coconut oil
- 1 tablespoon Chia seeds, soaked
- 4-5 ice cubes

Directions:
1. To make this smoothie, add the greens and the fruits to your blender jar and process it for 30 seconds on high.
2. Next add the water, ice cubes, yogurt and Chia seeds and blend for 30 seconds.
3. Lastly add the coconut oil and whizz up on high for 30 seconds more.
4. Pour into glasses and serve immediately.

Nutrition Info: (Per Serving): Calories- 233, Fat- 5 g, Protein- 4 g, Carbohydrates- 50 g

Banana-beet Smoothie

Servings: 2
Cooking Time: 5 Minutes
Ingredients:
- 1 cup whole strawberries (fresh or frozen)
- 1 large red beet, peeled and chipped
- 1 large banana (fresh or frozen)
- 1 orange, peeled and de seeded
- 2 cups fresh spinach
- 1 cup fresh kale, stems removed

- 1 cup unsweetened almond milk

Directions:
1. Add everything to the blender jar, secure the lid and pulse until thick and creamy.

Nutrition Info: (Per Serving): Calories- 333, Fat- 4 g, Protein- 10 g, Carbohydrates- 71 g

Strawberry-chia Smoothie

Servings: 2
Cooking Time: 2 Minutes
Ingredients:
- 1 ½ cups whole strawberries (fresh or frozen)
- 2 medium bananas, fresh or frozen
- 1 cup unsweetened almond milk
- 2 tablespoon Chia seeds, soaked
- 3-4 fresh collard leaves, stems removed
- 2-3 ice cubes (optional)

Directions:
1. Add all the ingredients into your blender and whip it up until the smoothie is thick and frothy.

Nutrition Info: (Per Serving): Calories- 340, Fat- 0 g, Protein- 10 g, Carbohydrates- 65 g

Verry-berry Carrot Delight

Servings: 2
Cooking Time: 2 Minutes
Ingredients:
- 1 cup mixed berries
- ½ cup plain yogurt
- 1 cup almond milk
- 1 carrot, peeled and chopped
- A pinch or cinnamon powder

Directions:
1. Place all the ingredients in your blender and process it for 45 seconds.
2. Serve and enjoy immediately.

Nutrition Info: (Per Serving): Calories-159, Fat-3.5 g, Protein-8 g, Carbohydrates-24 g

OVERALL HEALTH AND WELLNESS SMOOTHIES

Lychee Green Smoothie

Servings: 2
Cooking Time: 2 Minutes
Ingredients:
- 1/3 cup baby spinach
- ½ cup cantaloupe, peeled and chopped
- ½ cup grapes, deseeded
- 3-4 lychees, peeled and pitted
- 1 cup filtered water
- 1 teaspoon freshly squeezed lemon juice
- ½ teaspoon freshly grated ginger
- 3-4 ice cubes

Directions:
1. Just place all the ingredients into the blender and pulse until smooth. Serve immediately!

Nutrition Info: (Per Serving): Calories- 77, Fat- 0.7 g, Protein- 1.9 g, Carbohydrates- 20 g

Pear-simmon Smoothie

Servings: 4
Cooking Time: 5 Minutes
Ingredients:
- 4 persimmons, chopped
- 2 small apples, cored and chopped
- 2 small pears, cored and chopped
- 2 handfuls of baby spinach
- 2 cups of mixed greens
- 1 cup filtered water
- 2 teaspoons of freshly squeezed lemon juice
- 4-5 ice cubes

Directions:
1. Place all the above ingredients into the blender jar and process until the mixture is thick and creamy.

Nutrition Info: (Per Serving): Calories- 239, Fat- 1 g, Protein- 3 g, Carbohydrates- 63 g

Dragon- Berry Smoothie

Servings: 3
Cooking Time: 5 Minutes
Ingredients:
- ½ cup dragon fruits, peeled and chopped
- ½ cup raspberries (fresh or frozen)
- ½ cup spinach, chopped and washed
- ½ cup mixed greens, washed and chopped
- 1 ripe banana, chopped
- 1-2 dates, pitted
- 1 ½ cups homemade almond milk
- A pinch of cinnamon powder

Directions:
1. To your high speed blender, add all the above mentioned items and process on high for 30 seconds. Pour into serving glasses and enjoy immediately.

Nutrition Info: (Per Serving): Calories- 320, Fat-7.4 g, Protein- 5 g, Carbohydrates- 62 g

Rasp-ricot Smoothie

Servings: 2-3
Cooking Time: 5 Minutes
Ingredients:
- 1 ½ cups whole raspberries (fresh or frozen)
- 1 cup low fat plain yogurt
- 2 apricots, pitted and chopped
- 3 teaspoons flax seed powder
- 3 tablespoon raw organic honey
- 4 teaspoons freshly squeezed lemon juice
- 4-5 ice cubes

Directions:
1. Place all the above ingredients into the blender jar and process until the mixture is thick and creamy.

Nutrition Info: (Per Serving): Calories-289, Fat- 3.5 g. Protein- 12.5 g, Carbohydrates-60 g

Fruit Bomb Smoothie

Servings: 2
Cooking Time: 5 Minutes
Ingredients:
- ½ cup whole strawberries (fresh or frozen)
- 2 tablespoons chopped kiwi fruit
- ¼ cup freshly prepared orange juice
- ¼ cup blueberries (fresh or frozen)
- 1 small banana, chopped
- ½ cup low fat plain yogurt
- ½ peach, pitted
- 3-4 ice cubes
- 1 teaspoon freshly squeezed lemon juice

Directions:
1. Whizz all the ingredients in the blender until smooth and serve.

Nutrition Info: (Per Serving): Calories- 136, Fat- 1 g, Protein- 3.5 g, Carbohydrates-30 g

Cherry- Date Plum Smoothie

Servings: 2
Cooking Time: 5 Minutes
Ingredients:
- ½ cup cherries, pitted
- 1 zucchini, deseeded and chopped
- 1 plum, pitted and chopped

- 1 teaspoon flax seed powder
- 1-2 dates, pitted
- 1 cup filtered water
- 1 teaspoon freshly squeezed lemon juice
- 3-4 ice

Directions:
1. Whizz all the ingredients in the blender until smooth and serve.

Nutrition Info: (Per Serving): Calories- 100, Fat- 0.5 g, Protein- 1.8 g, Carbohydrates- 25 g

Avocado- Citrus Blast

Servings: 2-3
Cooking Time: 5 Minutes
Ingredients:
- 1 small tangerine, peeled and deseeded
- ½ cup plain low fat yogurt
- ¼ cup mixed berries
- 1 tablespoon avocado flesh
- 1 tablespoon freshly squeezed lemon juice
- 2 tablespoon freshly squeezed lime juice
- 1 teaspoon flax seed powder
- 2-3 drops vanilla extract
- ½ teaspoon raw organic honey
- 3-4 ice cubes

Directions:
1. Place all the above ingredients into the blender jar and process until the mixture is thick and creamy.

Nutrition Info: (Per Serving): Calories- 245, Fat- 11 g, Protein- 11 g, Carbohydrates- 33 g

Yogi- Banana Agave Smoothie

Servings: 2-3
Cooking Time: 5 Minutes
Ingredients:
- 2 cups plain fat free yogurt
- 2 ripe bananas, chopped
- 3 teaspoon light colored agave nectar
- 2/3 cup blue berries (fresh or frozen)
- 3-4 ice cubes

Directions:
1. Pour all the ingredients into your blender and process until smooth.

Nutrition Info: (Per Serving): Calories- 275, Fat- 0.6 g, Protein- 11. 5 g. Carbohydrates-c66 g

Water-mato Green Smoothie

Servings: 2
Cooking Time: 2 Minutes
Ingredients:

- 1 cup watermelon, chopped (seedless)
- ½ cup whole strawberries (fresh or frozen)
- 1 cup mixed greens, washed and chopped
- ¼ cup vine tomatoes
- 2 teaspoon freshly squeezed lemon juice
- ¼ cup filtered water
- 2-3 ice cubes

Directions:
1. Whizz up all the above listed ingredients in your blender for 20 seconds and serve. Enjoy immediately.

Nutrition Info: (Per Serving): Calories- 160, Fat- 0.7 g, Protein- 4.5 g, Carbohydrates- 27 g

Citrus Coconut Punch

Servings: 2-3
Cooking Time: 5 Minutes
Ingredients:
- 1 yellow grapefruit, peeled and deseeded
- 2 mandarins, peeled and deseeded
- 1 large lime, peeled and deseeded
- Freshly squeezed juice of 1 lemon
- 2 cups fresh coconut water
- 1 teaspoon freshly grated ginger
- 4-5 ice cubes

Directions:
1. Load all the ingredients into your blender and whizz until smooth.

Nutrition Info: (Per Serving): Calories- 211, Fat- 0.6 g, Protein- 4.2 g, Carbohydrates- 53 g

Blue Dragon Smoothie

Servings: 2
Cooking Time: 5 Minutes
Ingredients:
- ½ cup unsweetened almond milk
- ½ cup dragon fruits, peeled and chopped
- A handful of blueberries (fresh or frozen)
- A handful of fresh kale
- A handful of baby spinach
- 1 tablespoon Chia seeds, soaked
- 3-4 ice cubes

Directions:
1. Add all the above ingredients into your blender jar and pulse until thick and frothy.

Nutrition Info: (Per Serving): Calories- 135, Fat- 2.3 g, Protein- 4.8 g, Carbohydrates- 22g

Berry-ssimon Carrot Smoothie

Servings: 3
Cooking Time: 5 Minutes

Ingredients:
- ½ cup fresh coconut milk
- 1 persimmon, pitted and chopped
- ½ cup blackberries (fresh or frozen)
- 1 cup baby spinach, washed and chopped
- A small handful of fresh kale
- 1 small banana, sliced
- 1 small carrot, peeled and chopped
- 3-4 ice cubes

Directions:
1. To you blender, add all the above ingredient and pulse until smooth.

Nutrition Info: (Per Serving): Calories- 350, Fat- 6.8 g, Protein- 9.2 g, Carbohydrates- 75 g

Mp3 Smoothie

Servings: 2
Cooking Time: 2 Minutes
Ingredients:
- 1 cup papaya, peeled, deseeded and chopped
- 1 large pear, cored and chopped
- 1 cup peaches (fresh or frozen)
- ½ cup plain low fat yogurt
- 1 ½ teaspoon flax seed powder
- 1 teaspoon freshly grated ginger
- 5-6 fresh mint leaves
- 4-5 ice cubes

Directions:
1. To you blender, add all the above ingredient and pulse until smooth.

Nutrition Info: (Per Serving): Calories- 111, Fat- 2.3 g, Protein- 4.7 g, Carbohydrates- 20 g

Date "n" Banana Smoothie

Servings: 2 Small
Cooking Time: X
Ingredients:
- 1 large banana, chopped (fresh or frozen)
- 2/3 cup low fat plain yogurt
- 5 medjool dates, pitted
- 1/3 teaspoon nutmeg powder
- 1 teaspoon Chia seeds, soaked
- ½ cup ice cubes

Directions:
1. Pour all the ingredients into your blender and process until smooth.

Nutrition Info: (Per Serving): Calories- 290, Fat- 1.6 g, Protein- 5.2 g, Carbohydrates- 70 g

Red Healing Potion

Servings: 3
Cooking Time: 5 Minutes
Ingredients:
- 2 cups fresh coconut water
- 1 ½ cup pomegranate seeds
- 1 ¼ cup of red grapes, deseeded
- 1 cup whole strawberries (fresh or frozen)
- 2 tablespoons freshly squeezed lemon juice
- 4-5 ice cubes

Directions:
1. Place everything in your blender jar and whizz until smooth and frothy.

Nutrition Info: (Per Serving): Calories- 182, Fat-1.2 g, Protein- 4.3 g, Carbohydrates- 44 g

Blueberry Cherry Wellness Potion

Servings: 2
Cooking Time: 5 Minutes
Ingredients:
- ¼ cup plain fat free yogurt
- 1/2 cup whole blueberries (fresh or frozen)
- ½ cups cherries, pitted
- A handful of strawberries (fresh or frozen)
- 1 tablespoon fresh avocado flesh
- 1 tablespoon wheatgrass powder
- 1 tablespoon flax seed powder
- 1 tablespoon freshly squeezed lemon juice
- 3-4 ice cubes

Directions:
1. To you blender, add all the above ingredient and pulse until smooth.

Nutrition Info: (Per Serving): Calories- 155, Fat- 5.5 g, Protein- 6.2 g, Carbohydrates- 24 g

Apple Cucumber

Servings: 2-3
Cooking Time: 5 Minutes
Ingredients:
- 1 green apple, cored and chopped
- 1 green cucumber, deseeded and chopped
- 1/3 cup collard greens, chopped
- 1 ½ teaspoons Chia seeds, soaked
- 1 tablespoon freshly squeezed lemon juice
- 5-6 fresh mint leaves
- 1 cup filtered water
- 3-4 ice cubes

Directions:
1. Add all the above ingredients into your blender jar and pulse until thick and frothy.

Nutrition Info: (Per Serving): Calories- 114, Fat- 3.2 g, Protein- 3.1 g, Carbohydrates- 25 g

Mango Cantaloupe Smoothie

Servings: 2
Cooking Time: 2 Minutes
Ingredients:
- ½ cup mango, peeled and chopped
- ½ cup cantaloupe, peeled and chopped
- ¼ cup pineapple, peeled and chopped
- ¼ cup unsweetened almond milk
- 2 tablespoons almond flakes
- 1 tablespoon freshly squeezed lemon juice
- 3-4 ice cubes

Directions:
1. Dump all the ingredients into the blender and whip it up until the smoothie is thick and creamy.

Nutrition Info: (Per Serving): Calories- 152, Fat- 6.9 g, Protein- 4.3 g, Carbohydrates- 23 g

Orange Cranberry Smoothie

Servings: 2
Cooking Time: 5 Minutes
Ingredients:
- 1 cup cranberries (fresh or frozen)
- 2/3 cup plain low fat yogurt
- ½ teaspoon vanilla extract
- ½ cup freshly prepared orange juice
- 1 tablespoon raw organic honey
- 1 tablespoon wheat germ
- 5-6 ice cubes

Directions:
1. Place all the above ingredients into the blender jar and process until the mixture is thick and creamy.

Nutrition Info: (Per Serving): Calories- 255, Fat- 1.4 g, Protein- 7.2 g, Carbohydrates- 55 g

Finana Smoothie

Servings: 2
Cooking Time: 5 Minutes
Ingredients:
- 1 banana, chopped (fresh or frozen)
- 2 figs, chopped
- A handful of mixed greens, washed
- ½ cup filtered water
- 1 teaspoon raw organic honey
- 2-3 ice cubes

Directions:
1. Load your blender with all the ingredients and puree until smoothie is thick and creamy.

Nutrition Info: (Per Serving): Calories- 330, Fat- 1.7 g, Protein- 5.5 g, Carbohydrates- 87 g

Apple Blackberry Wonder

Servings: 2
Cooking Time: 2 Minutes
Ingredients:
- 1 cup blackberries (fresh or frozen)
- ½ cup fat free plain yogurt
- 1 tablespoon raw organic honey
- ½ cup freshly prepared apple juice
- ½ banana, sliced
- 2 teaspoon freshly squeezed lemon juice
- 3-4 ice cubes

Directions:
1. Add all the above listed items into the blender and blend until well combined.

Nutrition Info: (Per Serving): Calories- 260, Fat- 0.9 g, Protein- 5.5 g, Carbohydrates- 64 g

Trimelon Melba

Servings: 3
Cooking Time: 5 Minutes
Ingredients:
- 1 ¼ cups watermelon, chopped (seedless)
- ½ cup honeydew melon, chopped
- 1 ¼ cup cantaloupe, chopped
- 1 teaspoon raw organic honey
- 2-3 mint leaves
- ¼ cup freshly squeezed orange juice
- 3-4 ice cubes

Directions:
1. Dump all the ingredients into the blender and whip it up until the smoothie is thick and creamy.

Nutrition Info: (Per Serving): Calories-100, Fat- 0.6 g, Protein- 1.9 g, Carbohydrates- 25 g

Drink Your Salad Smoothie

Servings: 2
Cooking Time: 5 Minutes
Ingredients:
- 4 vine tomatoes, washed
- 1 teaspoon avocado flesh
- 1 red bell pepper, deseeded
- ½ green zucchini, chopped
- 3-4 celery stalks, chopped
- ¼ white onion
- 1 teaspoon of flax seed powder
- A pinch of cayenne pepper
- A pinch of paprika or chili powder
- ¼ cup filtered water

Directions:

1. Dump all the ingredients into the blender and whip it up until the smoothie is thick and creamy.
Nutrition Info: (Per Serving): Calories-458, Fat- 16.5 g, Protein- 16.8 g, Carbohydrates- 78 g

Chia Mango-nut Smoothie

Servings: 2
Cooking Time: 5 Minutes
Ingredients:
- 1 cup fresh coconut milk
- 1 cup mango, chopped
- 1 tablespoons Chia seeds
- 2 teaspoons freshly squeezed lemon juice
- 2 teaspoons freshly squeezed lime juice
- 2 teaspoons raw organic honey
- 6-7 ice cubes

Directions:
1. Dump all the ingredients into the blender and whip it up until the smoothie is thick and creamy.
Nutrition Info: (Per Serving): Calories- 211 g, Fat- 11 g, Protein-1.4 g, Carbohydrates-35 g

Nutty Apple Smoothie

Servings: 2
Cooking Time: 2 Minutes
Ingredients:
- 2 apple, cored and chopped
- 2/3 cup plain low fat yogurt
- ¼ cup toasted peanuts
- 3 teaspoons raw organic honey
- 1 teaspoon almond butter
- 3-4 ice cubes

Directions:
1. Pour all the ingredients into your blender and process until smooth.
Nutrition Info: (Per Serving): Calories- 291, Fat- 11g, Protein- 8.3 g, Carbohydrates- 48 g

Peachyfig Green Smoothie

Servings: 1 Large
Cooking Time: 2 Minutes
Ingredients:
- 1 peach, pitted
- 2 large figs, chopped
- A handful of mixed greens
- ½ cup filtered water
- 2 teaspoon freshly squeezed lemon juice
- 3-4 ice cubes

Directions:
1. Place all the ingredients into the blender, secure the lid and whizz on medium high for 30 seconds or until done. Serve immediately.
Nutrition Info: (Per Serving): Calories-195, Fat- 1.3 g, Protein- 4.5 g, Carbohydrates- 50 g

LOW FAT SMOOTHIES

Ginger Cantaloupe Detox Smoothie

Servings: 2
Cooking Time: 10 Minutes
Ingredients:
- 1 cantaloupe, sliced
- ½ inch ginger, peeled
- 1 tablespoon flaxseed
- 1 pear, chopped
- 1 cup of water
- 1 cup ice

Directions:
1. Add all the listed ingredients to a blender except the ginger
2. Blend until smooth
3. Then add ginger and blend again
4. Serve chilled and enjoy!

Nutrition Info: Calories: 85; Fat: 2g; Carbohydrates: 19g; Protein: 2g

Apple, Dried Figs And Lemon Smoothie

Servings: 2
Cooking Time: 5 Minutes
Ingredients:
- 2 medium apples
- ¼ lemon
- A pinch of Himalayan pink salt
- 1 fig, dried

Directions:
1. Wash the apples, remove the pit and then roughly chop them
2. Chop the dried fig
3. Toss the chopped apples and figs into your blender
4. Add lemon juice and stir
5. Add a pinch of Himalayan pink salt
6. Serve chilled and enjoy!

Nutrition Info: Calories: 120; Fat: 2g; Carbohydrates: 25g; Protein: 5g

Berry-beet Watermelon Smoothie

Servings: 3
Cooking Time: 5 Minutes
Ingredients:
- ½ cup fresh coconut water
- ¼ cup fresh coconut flesh
- 1 ½ cup fresh watermelon, chopped (seedless)
- 1 large handful of strawberries (fresh or frozen)
- 1/3 cup raw beets, peeled and chopped
- 1 tablespoon is freshly squeezed lemon juice
- 4-5 ice cubes

Directions:
1. Load your blender jar with the above listed items and process until smooth.

Nutrition Info: (Per Serving): Calories- 180, Fat- 6.8 g, Protein-3.2 g, Carbohydrates- 27 g

Banana- Cantaloupe Wonder

Servings: 4
Cooking Time: 5 Minutes
Ingredients:
- 2 small banana, chopped
- 4 cups ripe cantaloupe, peeled and chopped
- 1 cup plain non gat yogurt
- 1 teaspoon vanilla extract
- Pinch of cinnamon powder
- ½ cup freshly squeezed orange juice
- 1 teaspoon raw organic honey
- 3-4 ice cubes

Directions:
1. Place all the ingredients into your blender and run it on medium high speed for 1-2 minutes or until done.

Nutrition Info: (Per Serving): Calories- 360, Fat- 3 g, Protein- 15 g, Carbohydrates- 75 g

The Pinky Swear

Servings: 2
Cooking Time: 5 Minutes
Ingredients:
- 1 pack (3.5 ounces) frozen dragon fruit
- ¾ cup low-fat Greek yogurt
- 1 cup frozen pineapple
- 1 cup unsweetened coconut milk

Directions:
1. Add all the ingredients except vegetables/fruits first
2. Blend until smooth
3. Add the vegetable/fruits
4. Blend until smooth
5. Add a few ice cubes and serve the smoothie
6. Enjoy!

Nutrition Info: Calories: 200; Fat: 3g; Carbohydrates: 36g; Protein: 6g

The Great Shamrock Shake

Servings: 1
Cooking Time: 10 Minutes
Ingredients:
- 1 cup coconut milk, unsweetened

- 1 avocado, peeled, pitted and sliced
- 1 tablespoon pure vanilla extract
- 1 teaspoon pure peppermint extract
- Liquid stevia
- 1 cup ice

Directions:
1. Add all the listed ingredients into your blender
2. Blend until smooth
3. Serve chilled and enjoy!

Nutrition Info: Calories: 195; Fat: 19g; Carbohydrates: 4.4g; Protein: 2g

Chai Coconut Shake

Servings: 1
Cooking Time: 10 Minutes
Ingredients:
- ¼ cup shredded coconut, unsweetened
- 1 cup coconut milk, unsweetened
- 1 tablespoon pure vanilla extract
- 2 tablespoons almond butter
- 1 teaspoon ginger, grounded
- 1 teaspoon cinnamon, grounded
- 1 tablespoon flaxseed, grounded
- 5 ice cubes
- Pinch of allspice

Directions:
1. Add listed ingredients to a blender
2. Blend until you have a smooth and creamy texture
3. Serve chilled and enjoy!

Nutrition Info: Calories: 233; Fat: 20g; Carbohydrates: 5g; Protein: 4g

The Big Blue Delight

Servings: 2
Cooking Time: 5 Minutes
Ingredients:
- 1 tablespoon blue spirulina powder
- 1 tablespoon hemp seeds
- ¾ cup plain low-fat Greek yogurt
- 1 fresh banana
- 1 cup frozen blueberries
- 1 cup unsweetened vanilla almond milk

Directions:
1. Add all the ingredients except vegetables/fruits first
2. Blend until smooth
3. Add the vegetable/fruits
4. Blend until smooth
5. Add a few ice cubes and serve the smoothie
6. Enjoy!

Nutrition Info: Calories: 245; Fat: 6g; Carbohydrates: 43g; Protein: 8g

Pomegranate- Ginger Melba

Servings: 3
Cooking Time: 2 Minutes
Ingredients:
- 2 cups freshly prepared pomegranate juice
- 2 bananas, chopped (fresh or frozen)
- 1 cup low fat plain Greek yogurt
- 1 teaspoon freshly grated ginger
- 5-6 ice cubes

Directions:
1. Place all the ingredients into your blender and run it on medium high speed for 1-2 minutes or until done.

Nutrition Info: (Per Serving): Calories- 195, Fat- 2.2 g, Protein- 8 g, Carbohydrates- 40 g

Sage Blackberry

Servings: 2
Cooking Time: 5 Minutes
Ingredients:
- 1-ounce blackberries
- 3 tablespoons cashew
- 1 pear, chopped
- 4 ounces pineapple
- 3 sage leaves
- ½ teaspoon maqui berry powder

Directions:
1. Add all the listed ingredients to a blender
2. Blend until you have a smooth and creamy texture
3. Serve chilled and enjoy!

Nutrition Info: Calories: 154; Fat: 6g; Carbohydrates: 24g; Protein: 3g

A Batch Of Slimming Berries

Servings: 2
Cooking Time: 5 Minutes
Ingredients:
- 1 tablespoon chia seeds
- ¾ cup plain low-fat Greek yogurt
- 1 cup kale
- 1 cup frozen mango
- 1 cup frozen mixed berries
- 1 cup unsweetened vanilla almond milk

Directions:
1. Add all the ingredients except vegetables/fruits first

2. Blend until smooth
3. Add the vegetable/fruits
4. Blend until smooth
5. Add a few ice cubes and serve the smoothie
6. Enjoy!

Nutrition Info: Calories: 200; Fat: 5g; Carbohydrates: 30g; Protein: 8g

Cantaloupe Berry Blast

Servings: 2
Cooking Time: 2 Minutes
Ingredients:
- 1 cup cantaloupe, chopped
- 1 cup whole blueberries (fresh or frozen)
- ½ cup unsweetened almond milk
- 1 tablespoon Chia seeds
- 1 teaspoon, raw organic honey
- 2-3 ice cubes

Directions:
1. Load your high speed blender jar with all the ingredients and puree until thick and smooth.

Nutrition Info: (Per Serving): Calories- 120, Fat- 3.3 g, Protein- 3.5 g, Carbohydrates- 37 g

Mango-berry Smoothie

Servings: 3
Cooking Time: 5 Minutes
Ingredients:
- ½ cup low fat plain buttermilk
- 1 cup low pat plain yogurt
- ½ lb whole strawberries
- 1 cup mango, peeled and chopped
- 1 small banana, chopped (frozen)
- 1 teaspoon raw organic honey (optional)
- 3-4 ice cubes

Directions:
1. Add everything to your blender and pulse it on high for 20 seconds and your smoothie is ready. Enjoy!

Nutrition Info: (Per Serving): Calories- 180, Fat- 15 g, Protein-5.5 g, Carbohydrates- 36.5 g

Banana Orange Pina Colada

Servings: 4
Cooking Time: 5 Minutes
Ingredients:
- 1 ripe banana, chopped (fresh or frozen)
- 1 cup freshly prepared pineapple juice
- 1 cup plain low fat yogurt
- ¼ teaspoon vanilla extract
- 1 cup freshly prepared orange juice
- 2 teaspoons freshly squeezed lemon juice
- 3-4 ice cubes

Directions:
1. Combine all the ingredients in a blender jar and run it for 1 minute or until smooth and creamy.

Nutrition Info: (Per Serving): Calories- 145, Fat- 0 g, Protein- 3 g, Carbohydrates- 33 g

Ginger-mango Berry Blush

Servings: 2
Cooking Time: 2 Minutes
Ingredients:
- 1 large handful of whole strawberries (fresh or frozen)
- ½ cup mango, peeled and chopped (fresh or frozen)
- ¼ cup low fat plain yogurt
- ¼ cup filtered water
- 2-3 drops of vanilla extract
- ½ teaspoon freshly grated ginger
- 1 teaspoon raw organic honey (optional)
- 1 teaspoon freshly squeezed lemon juice
- 3-4 ice cubes

Directions:
1. Whizz all the ingredients until well combined and serve.

Nutrition Info: (Per Serving): Calories- 135, Fat- 1.1 g, Protein- 4 g, Carbohydrates- 35 g

Mango Passion Smoothie

Servings: 4
Cooking Time: 5 Minutes
Ingredients:
- 2 cups mango, chopped (fresh or frozen)
- 1 ½ cups plain nonfat yogurt
- ¼ teaspoon vanilla extract
- 1 cup freshly prepared passion fruit juice
- ½ cup filtered water
- 2 tablespoon freshly squeezed lemon juice
- 4-5 ice cubes

Directions:
1. To you blender, add the above ingredient and pulse until smooth.

Nutrition Info: (Per Serving): Calories- 290, Fat-2 g, Protein- 10 g, Carbohydrates- 61 g

Pumpkin- Banana Spicy Delight

Servings: 2
Cooking Time: 5 Minutes

Ingredients:
- 1 cup pumpkin, chopped
- 1 small banana, peeled and chopped (fresh or frozen)
- 6 ounces of low fat plain yogurt
- ¼ teaspoon vanilla extract
- ½ teaspoon pumpkin spice or all spice powder
- 1 teaspoon raw organic honey
- Handful of ice cubes

Directions:
1. Whizz all the ingredients until well combined and serve.

Nutrition Info: (Per Serving): Calories- 170, Fat- 5.2 g, Protein- 6.5 g, Carbohydrates- 35 g

A Peachy Perfect Glass

Servings: 2
Cooking Time: 5 Minutes
Ingredients:
- 1 cup skim milk
- 1 cup frozen peaches
- 1 fresh banana
- ¾ cup Siggi's vanilla yogurt
- 1 tablespoon hemp seeds
- Dash of ground cinnamon

Directions:
1. Add all the ingredients except vegetables/fruits first
2. Blend until smooth
3. Add the vegetable/fruits
4. Blend until smooth
5. Add a few ice cubes and serve the smoothie
6. Enjoy!

Nutrition Info: Calories: 208; Fat: 6g; Carbohydrates: 32g; Protein: 10g

Quick Berry Banana Smoothie

Servings: 4
Cooking Time: 5 Minutes
Ingredients:
- 1 ½ cups unsweetened almond milk
- 2 small bananas, chopped (fresh or frozen)
- 2 cups mixed berries (fresh or frozen)
- 3 teaspoons flax seeds
- 2 teaspoons freshly squeezed lemon juice
- 4-5 ice cubes

Directions:
1. Whizz all the ingredients until well combined and serve.

Nutrition Info: (Per Serving): Calories- 165, Fat- 3.2 g, Protein- 2.8 g, Carbohydrates- 29 g

Slim-jim Vanilla Latte

Servings: 2
Cooking Time: 5 Minutes
Ingredients:
- Dash of ground cinnamon
- 1 tablespoon chia seeds
- ½ cup unsweetened vanilla almond milk
- ½ cup leftover coffee
- 4 ice cubes
- ¾ cup Siggi's vanilla yogurt
- 2 fresh bananas

Directions:
1. Add all the ingredients except vegetables/fruits first
2. Blend until smooth
3. Add the vegetable/fruits
4. Blend until smooth
5. Add a few ice cubes and serve the smoothie
6. Enjoy!

Nutrition Info: Calories: 211; Fat: 4g; Carbohydrates: 40g; Protein: 7g

Orange Banana Smoothie

Servings: 2
Cooking Time: 10 Minutes
Ingredients:
- 4 oranges, peeled and seeded
- 4 bananas
- 1 2-inch piece ginger root
- 2 carrots
- 2 cups of water

Directions:
1. Add all the listed ingredients to a blender
2. Blend until you have a smooth and creamy texture
3. Serve chilled and enjoy!

Nutrition Info: Calories: 164; Fat: 0.4g; Carbohydrates: 28g; Protein: 7.6g

Cauliflower Cold Glass

Servings: 2
Cooking Time: 5 Minutes
Ingredients:
- ½ cup frozen cauliflower, riced
- ½ cup frozen strawberries
- ½ cup frozen blueberries
- ¾ cup plain low-fat Greek yogurt
- 1 fresh banana
- 1 cup unsweetened vanilla almond milk

Directions:
1. Add all the ingredients except vegetables/fruits first

2. Blend until smooth
3. Add the vegetable/fruits
4. Blend until smooth
5. Add a few ice cubes and serve the smoothie
6. Enjoy!

Nutrition Info: Calories: 204; Fat: 5g; Carbohydrates: 33g; Protein: 8g

The Big Bomb Pop

Servings: 2
Cooking Time: 5 Minutes
Ingredients:
- 1 tablespoon chia seeds
- ¾ cup plain low-fat Greek yogurt
- 1 cup frozen strawberries
- 1 cup frozen blueberries
- 1 cup unsweetened vanilla almond milk

Directions:
1. Add all the ingredients except vegetables/fruits first
2. Blend until smooth
3. Add the vegetable/fruits
4. Blend until smooth
5. Add a few ice cubes and serve the smoothie
6. Enjoy!

Nutrition Info: Calories: 198; Fat: 5g; Carbohydrates: 30g; Protein: 7g

Carrot, Watermelon And Cumin Smoothie

Servings: 2
Cooking Time: 5 Minutes
Ingredients:
- ½ cup carrot, chopped
- ½ teaspoon cumin powder
- 1 cup watermelon, seeded
- A pinch of Himalayan pink salt

Directions:
1. Add all the listed ingredients to a blender
2. Blend until you have a smooth and creamy texture
3. Serve chilled and enjoy!

Nutrition Info: Calories: 112; Fat: 1.2g; Carbohydrates: 23g; Protein: 6g

Lettuce -0range Cooler

Servings: 3
Cooking Time: 5 Minutes
Ingredients:
- 2 cups carrots, peeled and chopped
- 2 large Clementine's, peeled and seeded
- 1 cup romaine lettuce, washed and chopped
- 2/3 cup plain Greek yogurt (low fat)
- ¼ teaspoon vanilla extract
- 4-5 ice cubes

Directions:
1. Combine all the ingredients in a blender jar and run it for 1 minute or until smooth and creamy.

Nutrition Info: (Per Serving): Calories- 99, Fat- 0.2 g, Protein- 6 g, Carbohydrates- 20 g

Mini Pepper Popper Smoothie

Servings: 2
Cooking Time: 5 Minutes
Ingredients:
- 5 ounces mini peppers, seeded
- 4 ounces pineapple
- 1 orange, peeled
- 3 tablespoons almonds
- ½ lemon, juiced
- 1 cup of water
- 1 teaspoon rose hip powder

Directions:
1. Add all the listed ingredients to a blender
2. Blend until you have a smooth and creamy texture
3. Serve chilled and enjoy!

Nutrition Info: Calories: 190; Fat: 8g; Carbohydrates: 21g; Protein: 5g

ANTI-AGEING SMOOTHIES

Powerful Kale And Carrot Glass

Servings: 1
Cooking Time: 10 Minutes
Ingredients:
- 1 cup of coconut water
- Lemon juice, 1 lemon
- 1 green apple, core removed and chopped
- 1 carrot, chopped
- 1 cup kale

Directions:
1. Add all the listed ingredients to a blender
2. Blend until you have a smooth and creamy texture
3. Serve chilled and enjoy!

Nutrition Info: Calories: 116; Fat: 5g; Carbohydrates: 14g; Protein: 6g

Beets And Berry Beauty Enhancer

Servings: 2
Cooking Time: 5 Minutes
Ingredients:
- 1 teaspoon ginger, grated
- 2 tablespoons pumpkin seeds
- ¼ cup avocado, chopped
- ¼ cup beet, steamed and peeled
- 1/3 cup frozen strawberries
- 1/3 cup frozen raspberries
- 1/3 cup frozen blueberries
- ½ cup Greek yogurt
- ½ cup unsweetened almond milk

Directions:
1. Add all the ingredients except vegetables/fruits first
2. Blend until smooth
3. Add the vegetable/fruits
4. Blend until smooth
5. Add a few ice cubes and serve the smoothie
6. Enjoy!

Nutrition Info: Calories: 418; Fat: 20g; Carbohydrates: 50g; Protein: 17g

The Anti-aging Turmeric And Coconut Delight

Servings: 1
Cooking Time: 10 Minutes
Ingredients:
- 1 tablespoon coconut oil
- 2 teaspoons chia seeds
- 1 teaspoon ground turmeric
- 1 banana, frozen
- ½ cup pineapple, diced
- 1 cup of coconut milk

Directions:
1. Add all the listed ingredients to a blender
2. Blend until you have a smooth and creamy texture
3. Serve chilled and enjoy!

Nutrition Info: Calories: 430; Fat: 30g; Carbohydrates: 10g; Protein: 7g

A Honeydew And Cucumber Medley

Servings: 2
Cooking Time: 5 Minutes
Ingredients:
- 1 cup ice
- 1 Medjool date, pitted
- 1 tablespoon ground flaxseed
- 1 tablespoon coconut flour
- ½ lime, juiced
- 1 tablespoon fresh mint, chopped
- 1 cup honeydew
- 1 cup cucumber, chopped
- ¾ cup Greek yogurt

Directions:
1. Add all the ingredients except vegetables/fruits first
2. Blend until smooth
3. Add the vegetable/fruits
4. Blend until smooth
5. Add a few ice cubes and serve the smoothie
6. Enjoy!

Nutrition Info: Calories: 334; Fat: 7g; Carbohydrates: 50g; Protein: 20g

A Green Grape Shake

Servings: 2
Cooking Time: 5 Minutes
Ingredients:
- 1 cup ice
- 2 tablespoons chia seeds
- 1 orange, peeled and quartered
- 1 pear, cored and chopped
- 1 cup green seedless grapes
- 2 cups baby kale
- ½ frozen banana, sliced
- ½ cup silken tofu
- ½ cup of water

Directions:
1. Add all the ingredients except vegetables/fruits first

2. Blend until smooth
3. Add the vegetable/fruits
4. Blend until smooth
5. Add a few ice cubes and serve the smoothie
6. Enjoy!

Nutrition Info: Calories: 86; Fat: 8g; Carbohydrates: 3g; Protein: 2g

The Wrinkle Fighter

Servings: 1
Cooking Time: 10 Minutes
Ingredients:
- 2 brazil nuts
- 1 tablespoon flaxseeds
- 1 orange, peeled and cut in half
- 2 cups wild blueberries, frozen
- 2 cups kale, roughly chopped
- 1 ½ cups cold coconut water

Directions:
1. Add all the listed ingredients to a blender
2. Blend until you have a smooth and creamy texture
3. Serve chilled and enjoy!

Nutrition Info: Calories: 180; Fat: 15g; Carbohydrates: 8g; Protein: 5g

Maca – Mango Delight

Servings: 2
Cooking Time: 5 Minutes
Ingredients:
- 1 cup fresh coconut water
- 1 cup freshly prepared carrot juice or 1 ½ cup chopped carrot
- 1 large mango, peeled and chopped
- ½ teaspoon maca root powder
- ½ teaspoon cinnamon powder
- 1 teaspoon freshly squeezed lemon juice
- 3-4 ice cubes

Directions:
1. Into the blender jar, add all of the ingredients mentioned above and whizz until smooth.

Nutrition Info: (Per Serving): Calories- 220, Fat-0 g, Protein- 3 g, Carbohydrates- 10 g

Fine Tea Toner

Servings: 2
Cooking Time: 5 Minutes
Ingredients:
- ½ cup edamame shelled
- 1 cup dandelion greens
- 1 green apple, cored and peel on
- ½ frozen banana, sliced
- 1 cup brewed and chilled green tea
- 2 tablespoons walnuts
- 1-2 pitted Medjool dates
- 1 cup ice

Directions:
1. Add all the ingredients except vegetables/fruits first
2. Blend until smooth
3. Add the vegetable/fruits
4. Blend until smooth
5. Add a few ice cubes and serve the smoothie
6. Enjoy!

Nutrition Info: Calories: 490; Fat: 14g; Carbohydrates: 88g; Protein: 15g

The Feisty Goddess

Servings: 1
Cooking Time: 10 Minutes
Ingredients:
- 1 cup unsweetened almond milk
- 2 tablespoons lemon juice
- 2 tablespoons avocado, peeled and pit removed
- 1 tablespoon sunflower seeds
- ½ medium banana, ripe
- 1 cup packed spinach

Directions:
1. Add all the listed ingredients to a blender
2. Blend until you have a smooth and creamy texture
3. Serve chilled and enjoy!

Nutrition Info: Calories: 401; Fat: 42g; Carbohydrates: 4g; Protein: 2g

Simple Anti-aging Cacao Dream

Servings: 1
Cooking Time: 10 Minutes
Ingredients:
- 1 cup unsweetened almond milk
- 1 tablespoon cacao powder
- 6 strawberries
- 1 banana

Directions:
1. Add all the listed ingredients to a blender
2. Blend until you have a smooth and creamy texture
3. Serve chilled and enjoy!

Nutrition Info: Calories: 220; Fat: 9g; Carbohydrates: 20g; Protein: 6g

The Anti-aging Avocado

Servings: 2
Cooking Time: 5 Minutes
Ingredients:
- 1 cup ice
- 1 teaspoon vanilla extract
- 1 teaspoon grapeseed oil
- ½ cup avocado, chopped
- ½ cup of frozen strawberries
- ½ cup frozen peaches, chopped
- ½ cup plain Greek yogurt
- ¼ cup 100% pomegranate juice

Directions:
1. Add all the ingredients except vegetables/fruits first
2. Blend until smooth
3. Add the vegetable/fruits
4. Blend until smooth
5. Add a few ice cubes and serve the smoothie
6. Enjoy!

Nutrition Info: Calories: 447; Fat: 23g; Carbohydrates: 39g; Protein: 22g

The Anti-aging Superfood Glass

Servings: 1
Cooking Time: 10 Minutes
Ingredients:
- Water as needed
- ½ cup unsweetened nut milk
- 1-2 scoops vanilla Whey Protein
- 1 tablespoon unrefined coconut oil
- 1 tablespoon chia seeds
- 1 tablespoon almond butter
- ¼ cup frozen blueberries
- ½ stick frozen acai puree

Directions:
1. Add all the listed ingredients to a blender
2. Blend until you have a smooth and creamy texture
3. Serve chilled and enjoy!

Nutrition Info: Calories: 162; Fat: 14g; Carbohydrates: 10g; Protein: 3g

The Glass Of Glowing Skin

Servings: 1
Cooking Time: 10 Minutes
Ingredients:
- ½ avocado, sliced
- 2 cups kale
- 1 cup mango, chopped
- 1 cup pineapple, chopped
- 2 frozen bananas, peeled and sliced
- ½ cup of coconut water
- 1 tablespoon flax

Directions:
1. Add all the listed ingredients to a blender
2. Blend until you have a smooth and creamy texture
3. Serve chilled and enjoy!

Nutrition Info: Calories: 430; Fat: 40g; Carbohydrates: 20g; Protein: 10g

4 Superfood Spice Smoothie

Servings: 2
Cooking Time: 5 Minutes
Ingredients:
- 1 cup unsweetened almond milk
- 1 small banana, chopped (fresh or frozen)
- ¼ cup Goji berries
- 1 teaspoon cacao powder
- 1 teaspoon maca rot powder
- 1 teaspoon hemp seed powder
- 1 teaspoon Chia seeds, soaked
- ¼ teaspoon cinnamon powder
- ½ teaspoon raw organic honey
- 2-3 ice cubes

Directions:
1. Add all the ingredients into the blender and process until smooth and thick.

Nutrition Info: (Per Serving): Calories- 321, Fat- 15 g, Protein- 13 g, Carbohydrates- 42 g

Green Tea-cacao Berry Smoothie

Servings: 2
Cooking Time: 10 Minutes
Ingredients:
- 1 cup unsweetened almond or soy milk
- ½ cup strawberries (fresh or frozen)
- ½ cup blueberries (fresh or frozen)
- ½ cup raspberries (fresh or frozen)
- 1/3 cup freshly brewed green tea
- 1 tablespoon cacao powder
- 3-4 ice cubes

Directions:
1. To make the green tea, first takes a sauce pan, bring the water to a boil and take it off the heat.
2. Next add the green tea bag and allow it to steep it for 5 minutes.
3. Allow the tea to cool down to room temperature.
4. Then discard the tea bag.
5. Pour all the ingredients including the tea into the blender jar and run it on medium high for 30 seconds or until smooth.

Nutrition Info: (Per Serving): Calories-121, Fat- 2.4 g, Protein- 3.6 g, Carbohydrates- 21 g

Watermelon- Yogurt Smoothie

Servings: 2
Cooking Time: 5 Minutes
Ingredients:
- 2 cups watermelon chopped (fresh or frozen)
- ½ cup plain yogurt
- 1 tablespoon almond butter
- 1 teaspoon raw organic honey
- ½ teaspoon freshly grated ginger
- 4-5 ice cubes

Directions:
1. Add all the ingredients into the blender and pulse until smooth.

Nutrition Info: (Per Serving): Calories- 112, Fat- 1.7 g, Protein-4.4 g, Carbohydrates- 22.4 g

The Breezy Blueberry

Servings: 1
Cooking Time: 10 Minutes
Ingredients:
- Handful of mint
- 1 teaspoon chia seeds
- 1 tablespoon lemon juice
- 1 cup of coconut water
- 1 cup strawberries
- 1 cup blueberries

Directions:
1. Add all the listed ingredients to a blender
2. Blend until you have a smooth and creamy texture
3. Serve chilled and enjoy!

Nutrition Info: Calories: 169; Fat: 13g; Carbohydrates: 11g; Protein: 6g

Coconut Mulberry Banana Smoothie

Servings: 3
Cooking Time: 5 Minutes
Ingredients:
- 1 cup mulberries (fresh or frozen)
- 2 cups fresh coconut water
- 1/3 cup cranberries
- 1 large banana, chopped (fresh or frozen)
- 1 apple, cored and chopped
- 1 tablespoon hemp seeds
- 1 tablespoon flax seeds
- Freshly squeezed juice of ½ lime
- ½ cup ice cubes

Directions:
1. To your high speed blender, add all the items listed above and blitz until everything is well combined.

Nutrition Info: (Per Serving): Calories- 322, Fat- 15 g, Protein- 10 g, Carbohydrates- 70 g

The Super Green

Servings: 1
Cooking Time: 10 Minutes
Ingredients:
- 1 tablespoon agave nectar
- 1 bunch kale, spinach, Swiss chard or combination
- 1 bunch cilantro
- 2 cucumbers, chopped and peeled
- 1 lime, peeled
- 1 lemon, outer yellow peeled
- 1 orange, peeled
- ½ cup ice

Directions:
1. Add all the listed ingredients to a blender
2. Blend until you have a smooth and creamy texture
3. Serve chilled and enjoy!

Nutrition Info: Calories: 3180; Fat: 15g; Carbohydrates: 8g; Protein: 5g

Pineapple Basil Blast

Servings: 2
Cooking Time: 5 Minutes
Ingredients:
- 1 cup pineapple, peeled and chopped
- 1 cup fresh coconut water
- Freshly squeezed juice of 1 lime
- A handful if mixed greens of your choice
- A handful of sweet basil leaves
- ¼ cup baby spinach
- 1 cup cucumber, chopped
- 1 teaspoon raw organic honey
- 1 tablespoon freshly squeezed lemon juice
- 4-5 ice cubes

Directions:
1. Pour all the ingredients into the blender and process on medium speed for 45 seconds or until the desired consistency is reached.

Nutrition Info: (Per Serving): Calories- 153, Fat- 2.5 g, Protein- 4 g, Carbohydrates- 32 g

Dragon Fruit And Beet Smoothie

Servings: 3
Cooking Time: 5 Minutes
Ingredients:
- 1 medium dragon fruit, peeled and chopped
- 2 cups fresh coconut water
- ½ cup red beet, peeled and chopped
- ½ cup chopped lettuce
- ½ cup fresh arugula
- 1 large banana, chopped (fresh or frozen)
- Freshly squeezed juice of 1 lime
- ½ cup ice

Directions:
1. Load your high speed blender jar with all of the above listed ingredients and pulse until smoothie is well combined.

Nutrition Info: (Per Serving): Calories- 125, Fat- 0.6 g, Protein- 4.2 g, Carbohydrates- 31 g

Mango And Blueberry Bean Smoothie

Servings: 2
Cooking Time: 5 Minutes
Ingredients:
- 1 teaspoon ground flaxseed
- 2 tablespoons almonds
- ¼ cup kidney beans
- ½ frozen bananas, sliced into rounds
- ½ cup frozen mango
- ½ cup frozen blueberries
- 1 cup baby spinach
- ½ cup Greek yogurt
- ¾ cup water
- 1 cup ice

Directions:
1. Add all the ingredients except vegetables/fruits first
2. Blend until smooth
3. Add the vegetable/fruits
4. Blend until smooth
5. Add a few ice cubes and serve the smoothie
6. Enjoy!

Nutrition Info: Calories: 459; Fat: 10g; Carbohydrates: 73g; Protein: 26g

Date And Walnut Wonder

Servings: 1 Large
Cooking Time: 2 Minutes
Ingredients:
- 8-10 medjool dates, pitted
- 1/3 cup walnuts, halved
- 1 cup unsweetened almond milk
- 3 teaspoons cacao powder
- ½ teaspoon vanilla extract
- ¼ teaspoon cinnamon powder
- A handful of ice cubes

Directions:
1. Add everything into the blender jar, secure the lid and process until there are no lumps. Pour into glasses and serve.

Nutrition Info: (Per Serving): Calories- 230, Fat- 8.2 g, Protein- 7.9 g, Carbohydrates- 40 g

Ultimate Orange Potion

Servings: 2
Cooking Time: 5 Minutes
Ingredients:
- 1 large carrot, peeled and chopped
- 1 oranges, peeled and deseeded
- ½ cup mango, chopped
- 1-2 celery stalks, chopped
- 1 teaspoon freshly squeezed lemon juice
- ¾ cup filtered water
- 2-3 ice cubes

Directions:
1. Combine all the ingredients in a blender and process until smooth.

Nutrition Info: (Per Serving): Calories- 113, Fat- 1.1 g, Protein- 3.2 g, Carbohydrates- 26 g

Cacao- Goji Berry Almond Smoothie

Servings: 2
Cooking Time: 5 Minutes
Ingredients:
- 1 cup unsweetened almond milk
- 1 large banana, chopped (fresh or frozen)
- 3-4 fresh ale leaves, stems removed and chopped
- ¼ cup goji berries
- 2 teaspoons almond butter
- 2 teaspoon cacao powder
- 1/3 teaspoon cinnamon powder
- 4-5 ice cubes

Directions:
1. Load the blender jar with all the above listed ingredients and pulse on high for 30 seconds or until done.
2. Serve immediately.

Nutrition Info: (Per Serving): Calories- 345, Fat- 12 g, Protein- 13 g, Carbohydrates- 57 g

Acai Berry And Orange Smoothie

Servings: 2

Cooking Time: 5 Minutes
Ingredients:
- 1 cup Acai berry, fresh or frozen
- ½ cup pineapple, chopped (fresh or frozen)
- 1 cup whole strawberries(fresh or frozen)
- 1 cup freshly squeezed mango juice
- 1 banana, sliced (fresh or frozen)
- 1 teaspoon agave nectar or raw organic honey
- 3-4 ice cubes

Directions:
1. Load the blender with all the ingredients and process until the smoothie has reached your desired consistency.

Nutrition Info: (Per Serving): Calories- 201, Fat- 3 g, Protein- 3.1 g, Carbohydrates- 40 g

Natural Nectarine

Servings: 2
Cooking Time: 5 Minutes
Ingredients:
- 1 cup ice
- Pinch of turmeric
- 1 teaspoon vanilla extract
- 1 tablespoon coconut flour
- ¼ cup brazil nuts
- 2 cups baby spinach
- 1 nectarine, pit removed
- 1 cup seedless red grapes
- 1 cup coconut water

Directions:
1. Add all the ingredients except vegetables/fruits first
2. Blend until smooth
3. Add the vegetable/fruits
4. Blend until smooth
5. Add a few ice cubes and serve the smoothie
6. Enjoy!

Nutrition Info: Calories: 475; Fat: 22g; Carbohydrates: 53g; Protein: 11g

Super Duper Berry Smoothie

Servings: 2
Cooking Time: 5 Minutes
Ingredients:
- ½ cup unsweetened almond milk
- ½ cup frozen blueberries
- ½ cup whole strawberries (fresh or frozen)
- ¼ cup blackberries (fresh or frozen)
- ½ cup red cherries, pitted (fresh or frozen)

- 1 tablespoon cacao powder
- ½ cup romaine lettuce
- 1 teaspoon Chia seeds, soaked
- 1 teaspoon Spirulina powder
- 1 tablespoon hemp powder
- 2-3 ice cubes

Directions:
1. To make this smoothie, add all the ingredients into the blender and blitz for 45 seconds on medium high speed.
2. Pour into servings glasses and enjoy!

Nutrition Info: (Per Serving): Calories- 345, Fat- 20 g, Protein- 18 g, Carbohydrates- 75 g

Lychee- Cucumber Cooler

Servings: 3-4
Cooking Time: 5 Minutes
Ingredients:
- 1 ½ cup fresh coconut water
- 1 ½ cup red grapes
- 4-5 lychees, peeled and pitted
- 1 large cucumber, chopped
- 1 handful of spinach
- ½ cup of broccoli florets
- ½ cup chard or kale
- 1 tablespoon lemon juice
- 5-6 cubes of ice

Directions:
1. Place all the ingredients into your blender and run in high for 30 seconds or until smooth and frothy. Pour into glasses and serve immediately.

Nutrition Info: (Per Serving): Calories 272, - Fat- 1.6 g, Protein- 7 g, Carbohydrates- 70 g

Apple Kale Krusher

Servings: 2 Small
Cooking Time: 2 Minutes
Ingredients:
- ¾ cup unsweetened almond milk
- ½ cup fresh kale, stems removes and chopped
- 1 apple, cored and chopped
- ½ cup pineapple, peeled and hopped
- 3-4 ice cubes

Directions:
1. Just add all the ingredients into the blender and pulse until thick and smooth.

Nutrition Info: (Per Serving): Calories- 205, Fat- 2.4 g, Protein- 3.9 g, Carbohydrates- 61 g

DIGESTION SUPPORT SMOOTHIES

Cool Strawberry 365

Servings: 2
Cooking Time: 5 Minutes
Ingredients:
- 1 tablespoon chia seeds
- ½ cup water
- ¾ cup Siggi's whole milk vanilla yogurt
- 1 cup frozen peaches
- 1 cup baby spinach
- 1 cup frozen mixed berries
- 1 cup unsweetened vanilla almond milk

Directions:
1. Add all the ingredients except vegetables/fruits first
2. Blend until smooth
3. Add the vegetable/fruits
4. Blend until smooth
5. Add a few ice cubes and serve the smoothie
6. Enjoy!

Nutrition Info: Calories: 167; Fat: 6g; Carbohydrates: 25g; Protein: 8g

The Baked Apple

Servings: 2
Cooking Time: 5 Minutes
Ingredients:
- Dash ground cinnamon
- 1 tablespoon rolled oats
- 1 tablespoon hemp seeds
- ¾ cup Siggi's Whole milk vanilla yogurt
- 1 cup pear chunks
- 1 cup apple chunks
- 1 cup unsweetened vanilla almond milk

Directions:
1. Add all the ingredients except vegetables/fruits first
2. Blend until smooth
3. Add the vegetable/fruits
4. Blend until smooth
5. Add a few ice cubes and serve the smoothie
6. Enjoy!

Nutrition Info: Calories: 160; Fat: 4g; Carbohydrates: 33g; Protein: 2g

Pineapple- Flax Smoothie

Servings: 2
Cooking Time: 2 Minutes
Ingredients:
- 1 cup pineapple, chopped (fresh or frozen)
- 1 cup unsweetened almond milk
- 1 large banana, chopped
- 2 small kiwi fruits, peeled and chopped
- 1 teaspoon flax seed powder
- A pinch of cayenne pepper powder

Directions:
1. To your high speed blender jar, add all the mentioned ingredients and puree until smoothie is thick and creamy.

Nutrition Info: (Per Serving): Calories- 145, Fat- 2.1 g, Protein- 2.4 g, Carbohydrates- 36.1 g

Banana Oatmeal Detox Smoothie

Servings: 2
Cooking Time: 10 Minutes
Ingredients:
- 3 tablespoons collard greens
- 3 tablespoons oats
- 1 banana, peeled
- 1 apple, chopped
- 1 teaspoon cinnamon
- 1 cup ice
- 1 cup of water

Directions:
1. Add all the listed ingredients to a blender
2. Blend until you have a smooth and creamy texture
3. Serve chilled and enjoy!

Nutrition Info: Calories: 162; Fat: 1g; Carbohydrates: 41g; Protein: 3g

Mango-almond Smoothie

Servings: 3-4
Cooking Time: 5 Minutes
Ingredients:
- 2 large bananas, chopped
- 2 cups mango, chopped (fresh or frozen)
- 1 cup of unsweetened almond milk
- 1 cup coconut water
- 1 teaspoon raw organic honey
- 2 teaspoon of maca root powder
- 1 teaspoon flax seed powder
- 2-3 drops of vanilla extract
- 2-3 cubes of ice

Directions:
1. Load all the ingredients into the blender and whizz it for 30 seconds until smoothie is ready.

Nutrition Info: (Per Serving): Calories- 375, Fat- 8 g, Protein- 20 g, Carbohydrates- 75 g

Beet And Pineapple Smoothie

Servings: 2
Cooking Time: 5 Minutes
Ingredients:
- 1 large beet, peeled and chopped
- 1 cup pineapple, chopped (fresh or frozen)
- ½ cup parsley, chopped
- 1 teaspoon freshly squeezed lemon juice
- ½ teaspoon freshly grated ginger
- ¾ cup filtered water
- A pinch of Celtic salt

Directions:
1. Load your blender with everything listed above and whip it up on high for 20 seconds or until smooth.

Nutrition Info: (Per Serving): Calories- 100, Fat- 0.8 g, Protein- 2.8 g, Carbohydrates- 23.3 g

Pear And Avocado Smoothie

Servings: 2
Cooking Time: 5 Minutes
Ingredients:
- 1 cup plain yogurt
- 1/3 cup avocado, chopped
- 1 large pear, cored and chopped
- 3-4 sprigs of parsley
- 1 teaspoon freshly squeezed lemon juice
- ½ cup filtered water
- 3-4 ice cubes

Directions:
1. Pour all the ingredients into your high speed blender jar and process it for 30 seconds. Pour the smoothie into serving glasses and enjoy chilled.

Nutrition Info: (Per Serving): Calories- 220, Fat- 6.7 g, Protein- 8.1 g, Carbohydrates- 33 g

Tropical Storm Glass

Servings: 2
Cooking Time: 5 Minutes
Ingredients:
- 1 tablespoon hemp seeds
- ¾ cup plain coconut yogurt
- 1 fresh banana
- 1 cup unsweetened coconut milk
- 1½ cups frozen papaya blend (mix of papaya, mango, strawberry, and pineapple)

Directions:
1. Add all the ingredients except vegetables/fruits first
2. Blend until smooth
3. Add the vegetable/fruits
4. Blend until smooth
5. Add a few ice cubes and serve the smoothie
6. Enjoy!

Nutrition Info: Calories: 186; Fat: 0g; Carbohydrates: 14g; Protein: 1g

The Pumpkin Eye

Servings: 2
Cooking Time: 5 Minutes
Ingredients:
- Dash of ground cinnamon
- 1 tablespoon hemp seeds
- ½ cup unsweetened hemp milk
- ¾ cup Siggi's whole milk vanilla yogurt
- 1 fresh banana
- 1 cup kale
- 1 cup pure canned pumpkin

Directions:
1. Add all the ingredients except vegetables/fruits first
2. Blend until smooth
3. Add the vegetable/fruits
4. Blend until smooth
5. Add a few ice cubes and serve the smoothie
6. Enjoy!

Nutrition Info: Calories: 216; Fat: 3g; Carbohydrates: 48g; Protein: 3g

Spin-apple Pear Smoothie

Servings: 2-3
Cooking Time: 5 Minutes
Ingredients:
- 1 large banana, chipped
- 1 large apple, cored and chopped
- 1 pear, cored and chopped
- 2 cups baby spinach, washed and chopped
- 1 teaspoon raw organic honey (optional)
- 1 cup filtered water
- 2-4 cubes of ice
- A pinch of Celtic salt

Directions:
1. Combine everything in the blender jar and pulse until smooth and frothy.

Nutrition Info: (Per Serving): Calories- 73, Fat- 3 g, Protein- 4.2 g, Carbohydrates- 19.5 g

Noteworthy Vitamin C

Servings: 2
Cooking Time: 5 Minutes
Ingredients:
- 1 tablespoon chia seeds
- 1 clementine

- ¾ cup plain low-fat Greek yogurt
- 1 cup frozen strawberries
- 1 cup cantaloupe
- 1 cup unsweetened vanilla almond milk

Directions:
1. Add all the ingredients except vegetables/fruits first
2. Blend until smooth
3. Add the vegetable/fruits
4. Blend until smooth
5. Add a few ice cubes and serve the smoothie
6. Enjoy!

Nutrition Info: Calories: 209; Fat: 2g; Carbohydrates: 41g; Protein: 12g

Apple Chia Detox Smoothie

Servings: 2
Cooking Time: 5 Minutes
Ingredients:
- 3 tablespoons collard greens
- 1 mini cucumber
- 1 tablespoon chia seeds
- 4 kumquats
- 1 apple, chopped
- ½ teaspoon chia seeds
- 1 cup ice
- 1 cup of water

Directions:
1. Add all the listed ingredients to a blender
2. Blend until you have a smooth and creamy texture
3. Serve chilled and enjoy!

Nutrition Info: Calories: 108; Fat: 2g; Carbohydrates: 21g; Protein: 3g

Basic Green Banana Smoothie

Servings: 1
Cooking Time: 5 Minutes
Ingredients:
- 1 cup blueberries, frozen
- 1 cup almond milk
- 1 cup banana, frozen
- 1 cup spinach
- ½ tablespoon chia seeds

Directions:
1. Add all the listed ingredients to blender except kiwis
2. Blend until smooth
3. Add kiwis and blend again
4. Serve chilled and enjoy!

Nutrition Info: Calories: 146; Fat: 3g; Carbohydrates: 30g; Protein: 3g

Blueberry Chia Smoothie

Servings: 2
Cooking Time: 10 Minutes
Ingredients:
- 2 cups blueberries, frozen
- 1 cup coconut cream
- 4 tablespoons coconut oil
- 4 tablespoons swerve sweetener
- 4 tablespoons chia seeds, ground
- 2 cups full-fat Greek yogurt
- 2 cups almond milk, unsweetened

Directions:
1. Add all the listed ingredients to a blender
2. Blend until you have a smooth and creamy texture
3. Serve chilled and enjoy!

Nutrition Info: Calories: 351; Fat: 36g; Carbohydrates: 12.8g; Protein: 12.9g

Pineapple Yogurt Smoothie

Servings: 1
Cooking Time: 10 Minutes
Ingredients:
- 1 cup plain Greek yogurt, nonfat
- 1 cup apple juice, unsweetened
- 2 cups pineapple chunks
- 2 mangoes, peeled, pit removed and chopped
- 1 teaspoon chia seeds
- 16 ice cubes

Directions:
1. Add all the listed ingredients to a blender
2. Blend until you have a smooth and creamy texture
3. Serve chilled and enjoy!

Nutrition Info: Calories: 382; Fat: 1.6g; Carbohydrates: 88.5g; Protein: 11.2g

Yogurt And Plum Smoothie

Servings: 1-2
Cooking Time: 2 Minutes
Ingredients:
- 2 medium figs, chopped
- 2 plum, chopped
- 1 cup plain yogurt
- ½ teaspoon raw, organic honey
- 1 teaspoon freshly squeezed lemon juice
- ½ cup filtered water (or as needed)

Directions:

1. Add the fruits and liquids into your bender jar and whip it up until thick and frothy.
Nutrition Info: (Per Serving): Calories- 149, Fat- 1.9 g, Protein- 8.1 g, Carbohydrates- 26 g

Carrot And Prune Crunch

Servings: 2
Cooking Time: 5 Minutes
Ingredients:
- 2 cups unsweetened almond milk
- 1 cup carrot, peeled and chopped
- 1 large banana, chopped
- 4 tablespoons prunes
- 2 tablespoon walnuts
- 1 teaspoon vanilla extract
- 1/3 teaspoon cinnamon powder
- ¼ teaspoon nutmeg powder
- A handful if ice cubes

Directions:
1. Load everything into the blender and process on medium speed for 20 seconds until everything is well combined.
Nutrition Info: (Per Serving): Calories- 105, Fat- 4.7 g, Protein- 2.6 g, Carbohydrates- 15 g

Spin-a-banana Smoothie

Servings: 2-3
Cooking Time: 5 Minutes
Ingredients:
- 2 cups baby spinach. Washed
- 2 large bananas, chopped (fresh or frozen)
- 1 cup filtered water
- 2 teaspoons almond butter
- 1 teaspoon Chia seeds, soaked
- A pinch of cinnamon powder

Directions:
1. Place the ingredients in the blender jar, secure it firmly with the lid and run it on medium high until the smoothie is well combined without any lumps.
Nutrition Info: (Per Serving): Calories- 160, Fat- 5.3 g, Protein- 3.4 g, Carbohydrates- 30 g

Sapodilla, Chia And Almond Milk Smoothie

Servings: 2
Cooking Time: 5 Minutes
Ingredients:
- 4 medium sapodillas
- 2/3 cup almond milk
- 3 tablespoons chia seeds
- 1 tablespoon flakes

Directions:
1. Wash the sapodillas, peel them and then roughly chop them
2. Toss the chopped sapodillas into your blender
3. Then add almond milk
4. Add all the listed ingredients to a blender
5. Blend well and add almond on top
6. Serve and enjoy!
Nutrition Info: Calories: 113; Fat: 1g; Carbohydrates: 21g; Protein: 5g

Papaya- Mint Chiller

Servings: 2
Cooking Time: 2 Minutes
Ingredients:
- 1 ½ cups papaya, chopped (frozen)
- ½ cup plain yogurt
- 1 tablespoon regularly grated ginger
- 1 tablespoon of freshly squeezed lemon juice
- 1 teaspoon raw, organic honey or liquid Stevia
- 5-7 mint leaves
- A handful of ice cubes

Directions:
1. To your blender jar, add the ingredients one by one and process till you get a thick, creamy consistency.
Nutrition Info: (Per Serving): Calories- 177, Fat- 1.2 g, Protein-8.2 g, Carbohydrates- 41 g

Fine Yo "mama" Matcha

Servings: 2
Cooking Time: 5 Minutes
Ingredients:
- 2 teaspoons matcha powder
- 1 tablespoon hemp seeds
- ¾ cup coconut yogurt
- 1 fresh banana
- 1 cup frozen pineapple
- 1 cup unsweetened almond milk

Directions:
1. Add all the ingredients except vegetables/fruits first
2. Blend until smooth
3. Add the vegetable/fruits
4. Blend until smooth
5. Add a few ice cubes and serve the smoothie
6. Enjoy!
Nutrition Info: Calories: 216; Fat: 1g; Carbohydrates: 52g; Protein: 3g

Tomato- Melon Refreshing Smoothie

Servings: 2
Cooking Time: 2 Minutes
Ingredients:
- 1 large tomato, chopped
- 1 ¼ cup watermelon, chopped
- ½ small carrot, peeled and chopped
- 1 teaspoon hemp seeds
- ¾ cup filtered water
- 1 teaspoon freshly squeezed lemon juice
- 3-4 ice cubes

Directions:
1. Pour the above listed items into the high speed blender jar and pulse on high for 30 seconds. Pour the smoothie into serving glasses and consume immediately.

Nutrition Info: (Per Serving): Calories- 75, Fat- 1.6 g, Protein- 2.9 g, Carbohydrates-16 g

Mint-pineapple Cooler

Servings: 2
Cooking Time: 5 Minutes
Ingredients:
- 1 cup fresh coconut water
- 1 cup pineapple, chopped (fresh or frozen)
- 2 ripe bananas (fresh or frozen)
- 7-8 fresh mint leaves
- 1 teaspoon freshly squeezed lemon juice
- 4-6 cubes of ice

Directions:
1. To your blender jar, add all the ingredients and process for 45 seconds or until smooth.

Nutrition Info: (Per Serving): Calories- 150, Fat- 0.6 g, Protein- 2.6 g, Carbohydrates- 39 g

Almond And Date Smoothie

Servings: 2
Cooking Time: 5 Minutes
Ingredients:
- 1 cup unsweetened almond milk
- 3 teaspoons almond butter
- 2 cups baby spinach, washed and chopped
- 1 large apple, cored and chopped
- 1/3 teaspoon vanilla extract
- 2-3 medjool dates, pitted
- A pinch of cinnamon powder
- A pinch of Celtic salt
- 2-3 ice cubes

Directions:
1. Combine all the above listed items in the blender jar and whip it up nice and smooth. Pour into 2 servings lasses and enjoy.

Nutrition Info: (Per Serving): Calories- 500, Fat- 19 g, Protein- 11 g, Carbohydrates- 82 g

Coconut Berry Smoothie

Servings: 1 Large
Cooking Time: 5 Minutes
Ingredients:
- ½ cup coconut milk
- ½ cup coconut water
- 1 cup whole strawberries (fresh or frozen)
- 1 large banana, chopped
- 3 teaspoons hemp seed powder
- 1 teaspoon flax seed powder
- 1 teaspoon raw, organic honey

Directions:
1. Whizz up all the ingredients in your high speed blender for 30 seconds and serve immediately.

Nutrition Info: (Per Serving): Calories- 355, Fat- 11.5 g, Protein- 23 g, Carbohydrates- 47 g

The Nutty Macadamia Delight

Servings: 1
Cooking Time: 10 Minutes
Ingredients:
- Oz Macadamia nuts
- 1 cup spinach
- 1 tablespoon chia seeds
- 1 packet stevia, if you want
- 2/3 cup water
- ¼ cup heavy cream

Directions:
1. Add all the listed ingredients into your blender
2. Blend until smooth
3. Serve chilled and enjoy!

Nutrition Info: Calories: 485; Fat: 48g; Carbohydrates: 13g; Protein: 7g

Hearty Papaya Drink

Servings: 2
Cooking Time: 5 Minutes
Ingredients:
- 1 tablespoon chia seeds
- ¾ cup plain coconut yogurt
- 1 cup baby spinach
- 1 cup frozen papaya
- 1 cup frozen tropical fruit mix
- 1 cup coconut milk, unsweetened

Directions:
1. Add all the ingredients except vegetables/fruits first

2. Blend until smooth
3. Add the vegetable/fruits
4. Blend until smooth
5. Add a few ice cubes and serve the smoothie
6. Enjoy!

Nutrition Info: Calories: 192; Fat: 7g; Carbohydrates: 31g; Protein: 3g

Great Green Garden

Servings: 2
Cooking Time: 5 Minutes
Ingredients:
- 1 teaspoon spirulina
- Few fresh mint leaves
- ½ cup cucumber, peeled
- ¾ cup plain coconut yogurt
- 1 cup pineapple, frozen
- 1 cup mango, frozen
- 1 cup unsweetened coconut milk

Directions:
1. Add all the ingredients except vegetables/fruits first
2. Blend until smooth
3. Add the vegetable/fruits
4. Blend until smooth
5. Add a few ice cubes and serve the smoothie
6. Enjoy!

Nutrition Info: Calories: 200; Fat: 6g; Carbohydrates: 32g; Protein: 10g

The Amazing Acai

Servings: 2
Cooking Time: 5 Minutes
Ingredients:
- 1 tablespoon hemp seeds
- 1 pack frozen acai
- 1 cup baby spinach
- ¾ cup plain coconut yogurt
- 1 fresh banana
- 1 cup unsweetened hemp milk

Directions:
1. Add all the ingredients except vegetables/fruits first
2. Blend until smooth
3. Add the vegetable/fruits
4. Blend until smooth
5. Add a few ice cubes and serve the smoothie
6. Enjoy!

Nutrition Info: Calories: 225; Fat: 8g; Carbohydrates: 40g; Protein: 4g

Grape And Nectarine Blende

Servings: 1
Cooking Time: 5 Minutes
Ingredients:
- 1 cup red or green grapes, seedless
- 1 large nectarine, peeled and chopped
- 1 cup plain yogurt
- 1 teaspoon freshly squeezed lemon juice
- 1 teaspoon raw organic honey
- ¼ teaspoon cinnamon powder
- 1/3 cup filtered water

Directions:
1. To your high speed blender jar, add the ingredients and puree it until creamy and thick.

Nutrition Info: (Per Serving): Calories- 201, Fat- 2.2 g, Protein- 8.9 g, Carbohydrates- 32 g

ANTI-INFLAMMATORY SMOOTHIES

Guava Berry Smoothie

Servings: 2
Cooking Time: 5 Minutes
Ingredients:
- ½ guava, chopped
- 1 cup strawberries (fresh or frozen)
- 2 bananas (fresh or frozen)
- 4 cups spinach, washed
- 6 ounces of filtered water

Directions:
1. Load the blender with all the ingredients and whip it up for 1 minute until smooth.
2. Pour in a tall glass and enjoy!

Nutrition Info: (Per Serving): Calories-339, Fat 2g, Protein- 9.1 g, Carbohydrates-81 g

Pineapple & Coconut Smoothie

Servings: 1
Cooking Time: 10 Minutes
Ingredients:
- 1 cup fresh pineapple, diced
- 1 tablespoon coconut, shredded
- ½ lime, peeled and seeded
- 1 tablespoon chia seeds
- 1 teaspoon ground turmeric
- Pinch of freshly ground black pepper
- ½ cup coconut water

Directions:
1. In a high speed blender, add all ingredients and pulse till smooth.
2. Transfer into a glass and serve immediately.

Pineapple & Almond Smoothie

Servings: 3
Cooking Time: 10 Minutes
Ingredients:
- 1 cup fresh pineapple, peeled and chopped
- ¼ cup blanched almonds
- ½ cup fresh pineapple juice
- ½ teaspoon pure maple syrup
- ½ cup fresh pineapple juice
- ¼ cup rice milk
- ½ cup ice cubes, crushed

Directions:
1. In a high speed blender, add all ingredients and pulse till smooth.
2. Transfer into a glass and serve immediately.

Nutrition Info: (Per Serving):Calories: 96.7, Fat: 5.2g, Sat Fat: 0.5g, Carbohydrates: 11.6g, Fiber: 1.3g, Protein: 2.5g

Cherry & Blueberry Smoothie

Servings: 1
Cooking Time: 10 Minutes
Ingredients:
- 2 cups escarole
- ½ cup frozen blueberries
- ½ cup frozen cherries
- ¼ teaspoon ground cinnamon
- ¼ teaspoon ground turmeric
- 1 scoop of chocolate protein powder
- 1 cup filtered water
- 5 ice cubes, crushed

Directions:
1. In a high speed blender, add all ingredients and pulse till smooth.
2. Transfer into a glass and serve immediately.

Cherry & Pineapple Smoothie

Servings: 1
Cooking Time: 10 Minutes
Ingredients:
- ¼ of pineapple, peeled and chopped
- 12 fresh cherries, pitted
- ¼ of beetroot, peeled and chopped
- 1 tablespoon chia seeds
- 1 cup coconut water
- ½ cup ice, crushed

Directions:
1. In a high speed blender, add all ingredients and pulse till smooth.
2. Transfer into a glass and serve immediately.

Nutrition Info: (Per Serving):Calories: 250, Fat: 4.5g, Sat Fat: 1g, Carbohydrates: 51g, Fiber: 10g, Sugar: 30g, Protein: 6g, Sodium: 270mg

Pineapple & Mango Smoothie

Servings: 1
Cooking Time: 10 Minutes
Ingredients:
- 2¼ cups mixed mango and pineapple, peeled and chopped
- 1 tablespoon chia seeds
- 1 teaspoon ground turmeric
- ½ teaspoon ground ginger
- ½ teaspoon ground cinnamon
- Pinch of vanilla powder
- 1 cup coconut milk
- 1 teaspoon coconut oil

Directions:
1. In a high speed blender, add all ingredients and pulse till smooth.
2. Transfer into a glass and serve immediately.

Tangy Mango & Spinach Smoothie

Servings: 2
Cooking Time: 10 Minutes
Ingredients:
- 2 cups frozen mango, peeled, pitted and chopped
- 3 cups fresh spinach, chopped
- 1 teaspoon ground turmeric
- 16-ounce fresh coconut water
- 1 tablespoon lemon juice
- 1 tablespoon lime juice

Directions:
1. In a high speed blender, add all ingredients and pulse till smooth.
2. Transfer into 2 glasses and serve immediately.

Apple, Strawberry & Beet Smoothie

Servings: 4
Cooking Time: 10 Minutes
Ingredients:
- 2 cups frozen strawberries, hulled and sliced
- 1 beet, peeled and chopped
- 1 cup apple, peeled, cored and sliced
- 3 Medjool dates, pitted and chopped
- ¼ cup extra virgin coconut oil
- ½ cup unsweetened almond milk

Directions:
1. In a high speed blender, add all ingredients and pulse till smooth.
2. Transfer into a glass and serve immediately.

Nutrition Info: (Per Serving):Calories: 223.4, Fat: 14.6g, Carbohydrates: 22.3g, Fiber: 3.9g, Protein: 1.5g, Sodium: 49.7mg

Pineapple, Mango & Coconut Smoothie

Servings: 2
Cooking Time: 10 Minutes
Ingredients:
- 1 cup pineapple, chopped
- ½ cup mango, peeled, pitted and chopped
- Flesh and water of a coconut
- 1 tablespoon Goji berries
- ½ teaspoon fresh turmeric, chopped
- 1 teaspoon chia seeds
- 1 cup brewed green tea

Directions:

1. In a high speed blender, add all ingredients and pulse till smooth.
2. Transfer into 2 glasses and serve immediately.

Orange Squash Tango

Servings: 1
Cooking Time: 5 Minutes
Ingredients:
- 1 cup yellow squash, chopped
- 1 orange, peeled and copped
- 1 ounce kumquats (optional)
- 1 tablespoon hemp seeds
- ½ teaspoon freshly grated ginger
- 1 teaspoon freshly grated turmeric (or turmeric powder)
- 1 cup filtered water
- A few ice cubes

Directions:
1. Combine all the ingredients in a blender jar and run it for 1 minute or until smooth and creamy.

Chia And Cherry Smoothie

Servings: 1
Cooking Time: 5 Minutes
Ingredients:
- A handful of fresh cherries
- ½ cup of pineapple, cubed
- A couple of beetroot pieces
- 1 tablespoon of Chia seeds
- 2-3 ice cubes (optional)
- 8 ounces of coconut water
- 1 teaspoon of coconut oil

Directions:
1. Wash the cherries, pineapple and beetroot before chipping them and place in a blender.
2. Add the remaining ingredients to the jar and run it on high for 1 minute until smooth.
3. Serve chilled.

Nutrition Info: (Per Serving): Calories- 250, Fat-4.5 g, Protein- 6 g, Carbohydrates-51 g

Cherry & Kale Smoothie

Servings: 1
Cooking Time: 10 Minutes
Ingredients:
- 2 ripe bananas, peeled and sliced
- 1 cup fresh cherries, pitted
- 1 cup fresh kale, trimmed
- 1 teaspoon fresh ginger, peeled and chopped
- 1 tablespoon chia seeds, soaked for 15 minutes

- ½ teaspoon ground turmeric
- ¼ teaspoon ground cinnamon
- 1 cup coconut water

Directions:
1. In a high speed blender, add all ingredients and pulse till smooth.
2. Transfer into a glass and serve immediately.

Kale & Avocado Smoothie

Servings: 2
Cooking Time: 10 Minutes
Ingredients:
- 3 stalks fresh kale, trimmed and chopped
- 1-2 celery stalks, chopped
- ½ of avocado, peeled, pitted and chopped
- ½-1 ginger root, chopped
- ½-1 turmeric root, chopped
- 2 cups coconut milk

Directions:
1. In a high speed blender, add all ingredients and pulse till smooth.
2. Transfer into 2 glasses and serve immediately.

Watermelon, Berries & Avocado Smoothie

Servings: 1
Cooking Time: 10 Minutes
Ingredients:
- 1½ cups mixed frozen berries
- 1 cup watermelon, peeled, seeded and chopped
- ¼ of avocado, peeled, pitted and chopped
- 1-inch fresh ginger piece, peeled and chopped
- 2 teaspoons chia seeds
- ¾ cup fresh coconut water

Directions:
1. In a high speed blender, add all ingredients and pulse till smooth.
2. Transfer into a glass and serve immediately.

Cherry & Beet Smoothie

Servings: 1
Cooking Time: 10 Minutes
Ingredients:
- ¾ cup frozen pineapple, chopped
- 1 cup frozen berries
- ¼ cup frozen red beets, peeled and chopped
- ¼ small avocado, peeled, pitted and chopped
- 1 tablespoon chia seeds
- 1 teaspoon fresh ginger, peeled and chopped
- ½ teaspoon fresh turmeric, grated
- 2 teaspoon raw honey

- 1 cup unsweetened almond milk

Directions:
1. In a high speed blender, add all ingredients and pulse till smooth.
2. Transfer into a glass and serve immediately.

Mango- Papaya Blend

Servings: 2
Cooking Time: 5 Minutes
Ingredients:
- 2 cups papaya, chopped (fresh or frozen)
- ¾ cup mango, chopped (fresh or frozen)
- 1 cup unsweetened almond milk
- 1 teaspoon flaxseeds
- ¼ teaspoon vanilla extract
- A pinch of freshly grated lemon zest
- A pinch of cinnamon powder
- 2 teaspoon of freshly grated ginger
- 4-5 drops of raw organic honey
- 1 tablespoon freshly squeezed lemon juice
- A few ice cubes

Directions:
1. Place all the above listed ingredients into the blender jar and process until smooth.
2. Pour into glasses and enjoy!

Nutrition Info: (Per Serving): Calories-176, Fat-4.5 g, Protein- 2 g, Carbohydrates- 35 g

Pina-banana And Grapefruit Smoothie

Servings: 1
Cooking Time: 2 Minutes
Ingredients:
- 1 large banana, chopped (fresh or frozen)
- 1 cup pineapple, peeled and chopped
- ½ cucumber, chopped
- A handful of cilantro, washed and chopped
- ½ red grapefruit, peeled and chopped
- ½ cup of filtered water

Directions:
1. Place all the ingredients into the blender and BLEND! Serve immediately.

Nutrition Info: (Per Serving): Calories-262, Fat- 0 g, Protein-4 g, Carbohydrates- 66 g

Green Goblin Smoothie

Servings: 1
Cooking Time: 5 Minutes
Ingredients:
- 1 ½ cups of seedless green grapes
- ¼ cup freshly squeezed lemon juice

- ¼ cup avocado, chopped
- A handful of flat leaf parsley, washed and chopped
- 1 teaspoons freshly grated ginger
- 2-3 drops of raw organic honey or liquid Stevia
- 2-3 ice cubes

Directions:
1. Add all the ingredients into your blender and pulse for 1 minute and serve.

Nutrition Info: (Per Serving): Calories-244, Fat-6 g, Protein-4g, Carbohydrates-50 g

Strawberry & Kale Smoothie

Servings: 1
Cooking Time: 10 Minutes
Ingredients:
- ½ fresh strawberries, hulled and sliced
- 1 cup fresh kale, trimmed and chopped
- 1 celery stalk, chopped
- ½ of lime, peeled
- 1 cup coconut water

Directions:
1. In a high speed blender, add all ingredients and pulse till smooth.
2. Transfer into a glass and serve immediately.

Mango-pina Smoothie

Servings: 1
Cooking Time: 2 Minutes
Ingredients:
- 1 mango, chopped
- 1 cup of pineapple, cubed
- 1 handful of baby spinach
- 1 cup of filtered water

Dircctions:
1. Wash the pineapple and mango thoroughly before peeling and chopping into cubes.
2. Next, add all the ingredients into the blender and whir it up for 45 seconds to 1 minute until thick and frothy.

Nutrition Info: (Per Serving): Calories-219, Fat-0.8 g, protein- 3.9 g, carbohydrates -57.8 g

Ginger-carrot Punch

Servings: 1
Cooking Time: 5 Minutes
Ingredients:
- 1 carrot, peeled and chopped
- 1 small cup of pineapple, peeled and chopped
- A handful of spinach, washed

- ½ orange, peeled and deseeded
- 1 tablespoon Chia seeds (soaked)
- ¼ teaspoon freshly grated ginger
- ½ cup of filtered water

Directions:
1. Add the washed and chopped fresh produce into the blender jar.
2. Next add the Chia seeds and water and whip up the smoothie until there are no lumps.
3. Serve.

Nutrition Info: (Per Serving): Calories-337, Fat-0 g, Protein- 8 g, Carbohydrates-52 g

Coconut Carrot Pleasure

Servings: 1
Cooking Time: 5 Minutes
Ingredients:
- 1 small carrot, chopped
- 1 cup coconut water
- 1-2 peaches, fresh or frozen
- 1 small banana, fresh or frozen
- ¼ teaspoon freshly grated turmeric
- ¼ teaspoon freshly grated ginger
- 1 teaspoon coconut oil
- Few cubes of ice (optional)

Directions:
1. Place all the ingredients into the blender jar and process on high for 2 minutes or until done.

Nutrition Info: (Per Serving): Calories-220, Fats- 6 g, Proteib-4 g, Carbohydrates- 40 g

Spiced Banana Smoothie

Servings: 1
Cooking Time: 10 Minutes
Ingredients:
- 2 bananas, peeled and sliced
- 2 teaspoons ground ginger
- ½ teaspoon ground turmeric
- ½ teaspoon organic vanilla extract
- 1 tablespoon honey
- 1 cup coconut milk
- 6-8 ice cubes, crushed

Directions:
1. In a high speed blender, add all ingredients and pulse till smooth.
2. Transfer into a glass and serve immediately.

Pineapple & Watermelon Smoothie

Servings: 2
Cooking Time: 10 Minutes

Ingredients:
- 1 cup frozen pineapple, chopped
- 1 fresh orange, peeled and sliced (white pith and seeds removed)
- 2 cups frozen watermelon, peeled, pitted and chopped
- 1 teaspoon fresh ginger, peeled and chopped
- ½ teaspoon ground turmeric
- ½ cup coconut milk
- 1 teaspoon organic honey
- 1½ cups coconut water

Directions:
1. In a high speed blender, add all ingredients and pulse till smooth.
2. Transfer into 2 glasses and serve immediately.

Blueberry & Cucumber Smoothie

Servings: 1
Cooking Time: 10 Minutes
Ingredients:
- ½ cup cucumber, peeled and chopped
- ½ of small banana, peeled and sliced
- 1 cup frozen blueberries
- 1 tablespoon chia seeds
- 1 cup water

Directions:
1. In a high speed blender, add all ingredients and pulse till smooth.
2. Transfer into a glass and serve immediately.

Pear, Peach & Papaya Smoothie

Servings: 3
Cooking Time: 10 Minutes
Ingredients:
- ½ cup pear, peeled, cored and chopped
- ¾ cup peaches, pitted and chopped
- ¾ cup papaya, peeled and chopped
- 1 teaspoon fresh ginger, peeled and chopped
- 2 fresh mint leaves
- ½ cup coconut water
- 1 cup ice, crushed

Directions:
1. In a high speed blender, add all ingredients and pulse till smooth.
2. Transfer into 3 glasses and serve immediately.

Nutrition Info: (Per Serving): Calories: 48, Fat: 3g, Sat Fat: 0g, Carbohydrates: 12.5g, Fiber: 2.3g, Sugar: 8.8g, Protein: 7g, Sodium: 1mg

Pineapple & Green Tea Smoothie

Servings: 1
Cooking Time: 10 Minutes
Ingredients:
- 1 cup pineapple, chopped
- 1 small piece of ginger, peeled and chopped
- ½ teaspoon ground turmeric
- 1 teaspoon natural immune support
- 1 teaspoon chia seeds
- 1 cup cold green tea
- ½ cup Ice, crushed

Directions:
1. In a high speed blender, add all ingredients and pulse till smooth.
2. Transfer into a glass and serve immediately.

Peachy Ginger Smoothie

Servings: 1
Cooking Time: 5 Minutes
Ingredients:
- 1 cup unsweetened almond milk
- ½ cup peach (fresh or frozen)
- 1 small banana, hoped (fresh or frozen)
- ½ teaspoon finely grated ginger
- 1 teaspoon freshly grated turmeric
- ½ teaspoon hemp seeds
- 1 teaspoon cinnamon powder
- 1 teaspoon raw organic honey

Directions:
1. Whizz all the ingredients until well combined and serve.

Nutrition Info: (Per Serving): Calories-205, Fat-3.6 g, Protein-3.4 g, Carbohydrates- 44.7 g

Sweet And Spicy Fruit Punch

Servings: 1
Cooking Time: 10 Minutes
Ingredients:
- 1 cup freshly brewed green tea (room temperature or chilled)
- ½ cup papaya, chopped (fresh or frozen)
- ½ cup avocado, chopped
- ½ cup of blueberries (fresh or frozen)
- 1 tablespoon of Chia seeds
- A handful of baby spinach
- A pinch of cayenne pepper
- ½ teaspoon of freshly grated turmeric
- ½ teaspoon of freshly grated ginger
- ½ teaspoon of cinnamon powder
- 1 teaspoon of raw, organic honey
- 1 teaspoon of coconut oil

- A pinch of sea salt

Directions:
1. Brew a fresh cup of green tea and allow it to cool.
2. If you prefer chilled smoothie, refrigerate this tea for 1 hour.
3. Next, add all the dry ingredients into the blender and process until well combined.
4. Then, pour in the wet ingredients and blend it for 30 seconds more till the desired consistency is got.
5. Serve immediately.

Nutrition Info: (Per Serving): Calories 264, Fat 13 g, Protein- 4.1 g, Carbohydrates- 41 g

Sweet Potato & Orange Smoothie

Servings: 2
Cooking Time: 10 Minutes

Ingredients:
- 1 medium banana, peeled and sliced
- 1 cup sweet potato puree
- 1 teaspoon fresh ginger, chopped
- ½ tablespoon flax seeds meal
- 1 tablespoon almond butter
- ¼ teaspoon ground turmeric
- ¼ teaspoon ground cinnamon
- ¾ cup unsweetened almond milk
- ¼ cup fresh orange juice
- Ice, as required

Directions:
1. In a high speed blender, add all ingredients and pulse till smooth.
2. Transfer into 2 glasses and serve immediately.

MUSCLE, BONE AND JOINT SMOOTHIES

Strawberry-avocado Smoothie

Servings: 2
Cooking Time: 2 Minutes
Ingredients:
- 1 cup strawberries (fresh or frozen)
- ½ avocado, peeled, pitted and chopped
- 1 small pear, cored and chopped
- 1 small banana, sliced (fresh or frozen)
- 1 cup green lettuce (iceberg or romaine)
- ½ cup dandelion greens
- 1-2 chard leaves
- 1 cup filtered water
- 2-3 ice cubes

Directions:
1. Place all the ingredients in the blender and process until smooth. Serve chilled.

Nutrition Info: (Per Serving): Calories- 345, Fat- 7.9g, Protein- 5 g, Carbohydrates- 70 g

Orange Sunrise Smoothie

Servings: 3
Cooking Time: 5 Minutes
Ingredients:
- ¾ cup coconut water
- 2 large carrots, peeled and chopped
- 2 cups pineapple, chopped
- 1 cup freshly squeezed orange juice
- 1 cup lightly packed iceberg lettuce
- 2-3 celery stalks chopped
- 3 teaspoons Chia seeds, soaked
- ½ teaspoon freshly grated ginger

Directions:
1. To the blender, add all the ingredients and pulse until smooth.

Nutrition Info: (Per Serving): Calories- 345, Fat- 3 g, Protein- 7.5 g, Carbohydrates- 55g

Ginger- Papaya Smoothie

Servings: 2
Cooking Time: 5 Minutes
Ingredients:
- 1 cup plain yogurt
- 1 ¼ cup papaya, chopped
- 1 tablespoon raw organic honey
- ¼ teaspoon freshly grated ginger
- 1 teaspoon freshly squeezed lemon juice
- 4-5 ice cubes

Directions:
1. Add all the ingredients into the blender, secure the lid and pulse into smooth.

Nutrition Info: (Per Serving): Calories- 140, Fat- 3.4 g, Protein- 6.1 g, Carbohydrates- 25 g

Ginger- Parsely Grape Smoothie

Servings: 1
Cooking Time: 2 Minutes
Ingredients:
- 1 ½ cup red grapes, seedless
- ½ cup parsley, washed and chopped
- 2 tablespoons avocado flesh
- ¼ cup freshly squeezed lemon juice
- 1 teaspoon freshly grated ginger
- 3 drops of liquid Stevia or ½ teaspoon raw organic honey
- 4-5 mint leaves
- A handful of ice cubes

Directions:
1. Add all the ingredients into the blender and blitz until smooth.

Nutrition Info: (Per Serving): Calories- 230, Fat- 5.4 g, Protein- 3.9 g, Carbohydrates- 55 g

Orange Kiwi Punch

Servings: 2-3
Cooking Time: 5 Minutes
Ingredients:
- 1 cup freshly squeezed orange juice
- 1 cup mango, copped
- 2 kiwi fruits, peeled and chopped
- ½ cup arugula
- ½ cup ice berg lettuce
- 1 cup fresh kale, stems removed and chopped
- 1 teaspoon flax seed powder
- 3-4 ice cubes

Directions:
1. Place all the ingredients in the blender and process until your desired consistency has reached.

Nutrition Info: (Per Serving): Calories- 350, Fat- 2 g, Protein- 7g, Carbohydrates- 85 g

Banana- Guava Smoothie

Servings: 3-4
Cooking Time: 5 Minutes
Ingredients:
- 2 large bananas, chopped (fresh or frozen)
- ½ cup strawberries (fresh or frozen)
- ½ cup raspberries (fresh or frozen)
- 1 cup guava, peeled, deseeded and chopped
- 1 cup baby spinach

- ½ cup dandelion greens
- ½ cup romaine lettuce
- ½ cup water
- 1-2 ice cubes

Directions:
1. Pour all the ingredients into a high speed blender and process it on high for 20 seconds or until smooth and creamy.

Nutrition Info: (Per Serving): Calories- 325, Fat- 1.9 g, Protein- 10 g, Carbohydrates- 82 g

Apple –kiwi Blush

Servings: 2
Cooking Time: 5 Minutes
Ingredients:
- 1 cup unsweetened almond milk
- 1 large apple, cored and chopped
- 2 kiwi fruits, peeled and chopped
- 1 cup cucumber, chopped
- 2-3 collard green leaves, stems removed and chopped
- 3 teaspoons Chia seeds, soaked
- 2-3 ice cubes (optional)

Directions:
1. Place all the ingredients in a high speed bender and blitz on medium speed for 30 seconds or until smooth.

Nutrition Info: (Per Serving): Calories- 340, Fat- 0.5 g, Protein- 11 g, Carbohydrates- 60 g

Fruit "n" Nut Smoothie

Servings: 2
Cooking Time: 5 Minutes
Ingredients:
- 1 cup freshly brewed green tea
- 1 cup red cherries, pitted
- 1 cup whole strawberries (fresh or frozen)
- ½ kale, stems removed
- ¼ cup walnuts, halved
- ½ teaspoon freshly grated ginger
- 1 teaspoon wheat grass powder
- 1 teaspoon hemp powder

Directions:
1. Load all the ingredients in a high speed blender and process until it is smooth and thick.

Nutrition Info: (Per Serving): Calories- 255, Fat- 11 g, Protein- 8.9 g, Carbohydrates- 38 g

Kiwi Quick Smoothie

Servings: 2
Cooking Time: 2 Minutes
Ingredients:
- ½ cup unsweetened almond milk
- ½ cup plain yoghurt
- ¼ cup fresh coconut milk
- ½ cup whole strawberries (fresh or frozen)
- 1 kiwi, peeled and chopped
- 1 teaspoon raw, organic honey
- ½ teaspoon Chia seeds

Directions:
1. Combine all the ingredients in a high speed blender and process until smooth.

Nutrition Info: (Per Serving): Calories- 260, Fat- 9 g, Protein- 13 g, Carbohydrates- 37 g

Ginger Lime Smoothie

Servings: 3
Cooking Time: 5 Minutes
Ingredients:
- 1 cup fresh coconut water
- Freshly squeezed juice of 1 lime
- 1 cup pineapple, chopped
- 1 cup kale, stems removed and chopped
- ½ banana, chopped (fresh or frozen)
- ½ cup arugula
- 1-2 celery stalks, chopped
- 6-7 mint leaves
- ½ teaspoon freshly grated ginger
- 1 ½ teaspoon Chia seeds, soaked
- 2-4 ice cubes

Directions:
1. Place all the above listed ingredients into your blender and blend until smooth. Enjoy immediately.

Nutrition Info: (Per Serving): Calories- 345, Fat- 4 g, Protein- 8.5 g, Carbohydrates- 75 g

Spinach And Kiwi Smoothie

Servings: 2-3
Cooking Time: 2 Minutes
Ingredients:
- 1 cup fresh coconut milk
- 1 ½ cup fresh baby spinach
- ½ cup arugula, chopped
- 1 cup kiwi, peeled and chopped
- 1 small banana, chopped
- 1 teaspoon freshly squeezed lemon juice

Directions:
1. Add all the ingredients to a high speed blender and pulse until smooth. Pour into glasses and serve.

Nutrition Info: (Per Serving): Calories- 130, Fat- 2.1 g, Protein- 2 g, Carbohydrates- 29 g

Cilantro- Grapefriut Smoothie

Servings: 2-3
Cooking Time: 2 Minutes
Ingredients:
- 1 grapefruit, peeled and chopped
- ½ cup fresh cilantro, chopped
- 1 cup pineapple, peeled and chopped
- 1 small banana, chopped (fresh or frozen)
- 1 cup cucumber, chopped
- 1 tablespoon freshly squeezed lemon juice
- ¾ cup water
- 3-4 ice cubes

Directions:
1. To your high speed blender jar, add all the items mentioned above and process until the smoothie is thick and frothy. Pour into serving glasses and enjoy.

Nutrition Info: (Per Serving): Calories- 260, Fat- 0.2 g, Protein- 3.8 g, Carbohydrates- 68 g

Cucumber- Pineapple

Servings: 3
Cooking Time: 5 Minutes
Ingredients:
- 1 ¼ cups fresh coconut water
- 1 cup cucumber, chopped
- ½ cup pineapple, chopped
- 1 small avocado, peeled and chopped
- 1/3 cup fresh kale, stems removed
- 1/3 cup baby spinach
- ½ teaspoon freshly grated ginger

Directions:
1. Combine all the ingredients in a high speed blender and pulse until smooth.

Nutrition Info: (Per Serving): Calories- 260, Fat- 15 g, Protein- 7 g, Carbohydrates- 22 g

Pineapple Sage Smoothie

Servings: 2
Cooking Time: 5 Minutes
Ingredients:
- 1 cup pineapple, peeled and chopped
- 1 pear, core and chopped
- 2-3 sage leaves
- 1 teaspoon Chia seeds, soaked
- 1 teaspoon hemp seed powder
- 1 teaspoon freshly squeezed lemon juice
- ¾ cup water
- 2-3 ice cubes

Directions:
1. Add all the ingredients into the blender and run it on high for 30 seconds or until well combined.

Nutrition Info: (Per Serving): Calories- 250, Fat- 1.1 g, Protein- 5 g, Carbohydrates- 87 g

Berry-cantaloupe Smoothie

Servings: 3
Cooking Time: 5 Minutes
Ingredients:
- ½ cup whole strawberries (fresh or frozen)
- 1 cup mango, chopped
- 1 cups cantaloupe, chopped
- ½ cup fresh kale, stems removed
- 1 celery stalks, chopped
- 1 chard leaves, chopped
- A small handful of parsley
- ¼ cup baby spinach
- ½ cup filtered water

Directions:
1. Pour all the ingredients into a high speed blender and run in on high for 2 seconds or until the desired consistency is got.

Nutrition Info: (Per Serving): Calories- 375, Fat- 1.9 g, Protein- 6.8 g, Carbohydrates- 95 g

Orange Gold Smoothie

Servings: 2
Cooking Time: 5 Minutes
Ingredients:
- ½ cup fresh coconut milk
- ½ cup mango, chopped
- ½ cup pineapple, chopped
- ½ cup peaches, pitted
- ½ teaspoon freshly grated lemon zest
- ¼ teaspoon cinnamon powder
- ¼ teaspoon nutmeg powder
- ½ teaspoon cayenne pepper
- A pinch of Celtic salt
- ¾ cup filtered water
- A handful of ice cubes

Directions:
1. Place all the ingredients into the blender and whizz until thick and smooth.

Nutrition Info: (Per Serving): Calories- 171, Fat- 4.4 g, Protein- 2.9 g, Carbohydrates- 35 g

Cucumber- Pear Healer

Servings: 2
Cooking Time: 2 Minutes
Ingredients:
- 1 cup unsweetened almond milk
- 2 cups cucumber, chopped

- 2 large pears, cored and chopped
- 8-9 fresh mint leaves
- 1 teaspoon freshly squeezed lemon juice
- 1 teaspoon raw organic honey
- 3-4 ice cubes

Directions:
1. Just add all the ingredients into the blender and pulse until smooth.

Nutrition Info: (Per Serving): Calories- 285, Fat- 4.8 g, Protein- 5 g, Carbohydrates- 65 g

Coconut-blueberry Smoothie

Servings: 3
Cooking Time: 5 Minutes
Ingredients:
- 1 cup fresh coconut water
- 1 cup blueberries
- 1 large banana, sliced (fresh or frozen)
- 1 cup baby spinach, washed and chopped
- ½ cup fresh kale, stems removed and chopped
- ½ cup dandelion greens chopped
- 1 teaspoon freshly squeezed lemon juice

Directions:
1. Place all the ingredients into the blender and blitz until smooth.

Nutrition Info: (Per Serving): Calories- 250, Fat- 1.1 g, Protein- 4 g, Carbohydrates- 60 g

Maca –banana Smoothie

Servings: 2-3
Cooking Time: 5 Minutes
Ingredients:
- 1 cup fresh coconut water
- 1 tablespoon almond butter
- 1 ½ medium banana, chopped (fresh or frozen)
- ½ tablespoon maca powder
- ½ cup fresh baby spinach, washed and chopped
- 1 teaspoon Chia seeds
- A pinch of cinnamon powder
- 2-3 ice cubes

Directions:
1. Load the blender with all the ingredients and process on medium speed for 30 second or until smoothie is thick and creamy.

Nutrition Info: (Per Serving): Calories- 430, Fat- 19.8 g, Protein- 12 g, Carbohydrates- 58 g

SUPERFOOD SMOOTHIES

Tea And Grape Smoothie

Servings: 2
Cooking Time: 5 Minutes
Ingredients:
- 1 large apple, cored and chopped
- 1 cup red grapes, seedless
- ½ cup freshly brewed green tea (unsweetened and chilled)
- ½ cup plain low fat yogurt
- 1 teaspoons raw organic honey
- 1 teaspoons freshly grated ginger
- 3-4 ice cubes

Directions:
1. Load your high speed blender jar with all the ingredients and puree until thick and smooth.

Nutrition Info: (Per Serving): Calories- 131, Fat- 1 g, Protein- 5 g, Carbohydrates- 25 g

Basil- Bee Pollen Chlorella Smoothie

Servings: 2-3
Cooking Time: 5 Minutes
Ingredients:
- ½ cup pineapple, peeled and chopped
- 1 cup fresh coconut water
- 2 tablespoon ripe avocado flesh
- 1/3 cup low fat plain yogurt
- 1 teaspoon cacao powder
- 2 teaspoon coconut flakes
- 1 teaspoon raw organic honey
- 1 teaspoon bee pollen
- 1 teaspoon Chia seeds
- 1 teaspoon chlorella
- 1 teaspoon maca root powder
- 1 teaspoon freshly squeezed lemon juice
- 5-6 fresh basil leaves
- 1 teaspoon freshly squeezed lemon juice
- A pinch of Himalayan salt
- 4-5 ice cubes

Directions:
1. In a blender, combine all the above listed ingredients and blend until nice and smooth.

Nutrition Info: (Per Serving): Calories- 320, Fat- 14 g, Protein- 14 g, Carbohydrates- 40 g

Aloe Vera Smoothie

Servings: 3
Cooking Time: 5 Minutes
Ingredients:
- ½ cup pure aloe Vera gel
- ½ ripe avocado, peeled and pitted
- Freshly squeezed juice of ½ lime
- 1 ½ teaspoon pure coconut oil
- 1 cup mixed greens, washed and chopped
- 1 kiwi, peeled and chopped
- 1 teaspoon flax seed powder
- 1 teaspoon Chia seeds
- A pinch of Celtic salt
- 1 teaspoon raw organic honey
- 1 cup filtered water
- 4-5 ice cubes
- 1 teaspoon freshly squeezed lemon juice

Directions:
1. Add all the ingredients in the same order as listed above and blend until smooth and thick

Nutrition Info: (Per Serving): Calories- 360, Fat- 31 g, Protein- 3.2 g, Carbohydrates- 35 g

Berry Melon Green Smoothie

Servings: 3
Cooking Time: 5 Minutes
Ingredients:
- ¾ cup watermelon, chopped
- ½ cup whole strawberries (fresh or frozen)
- 1 ½ cup fresh baby spinach, washed and chopped
- 1 ripe banana, chopped
- 1 cup fresh coconut water
- Freshly squeezed juice of ½ lime
- 1 ½ teaspoon flaxseed powder
- 3-4 ice cubes

Directions:
1. Add all the ingredients in the same order as listed above and blend until smooth and thick

Nutrition Info: (Per Serving): Calories- 121, Fat- 1.5 g, Protein- 3 g, Carbohydrates- 25 g

Raspberry Carrot Smoothie

Servings: 2
Cooking Time: 5 Minutes
Ingredients:
- 1 large carrot, peeled and chopped
- 1 cup whole raspberries (fresh or frozen)
- ½ cup low fat plain yogurt
- 4 teaspoons Goji berries
- 1 tablespoon Chia seeds
- 1 tablespoon flaxseed powder
- 1 teaspoon raw organic honey
- 4-5 ice cubes

Directions:

1. To your high speed blender, add all the ingredients and pulse until smooth.
Nutrition Info: (Per Serving): Calories- 335, Fat- 12 g, Protein- 13.5 g, Carbohydrates- 45 g

Green Tea Superfood Smooothie

Servings: 4
Cooking Time: 5 Minutes
Ingredients:
- ½ cup freshly prepared pomegranate juice
- 1 cup freshly brewed green tea (unsweetened and chilled)
- ½ cup plain low fat Greek yogurt
- 1 cup mixed berries (fresh or frozen)
- 1 ripe banana, chopped (fresh or frozen)
- 1 large handful baby spinach, washed and chopped
- 1 teaspoon freshly grated ginger
- 1 teaspoon flaxseed powder
- 3-4 ice cubes

Directions:
1. To make this smoothie, add all the ingredients into your high speed blender and puree until smooth.
Nutrition Info: (Per Serving): Calories-130, Fat- 1 g, Protein- 6.9 g, Carbohydrates- 27 g

Chia Berry Spinach Smoothie

Servings: 2
Cooking Time: 2 Minutes
Ingredients:
- ½ cup whole strawberries (fresh or frozen)
- ½ cup whole blueberry (fresh or frozen)
- 1 cup baby spinach, washed and chopped
- ½ cup low fat plain yogurt
- ¼ teaspoons cinnamon powder
- 3 teaspoons Chia seeds, soaked
- 1 teaspoons flaxseed powder
- ½ teaspoons liquid Stevia or 1 teaspoon raw organic honey
- 4-5 ice cubes

Directions:
1. Pour all the ingredients into your blender and whizz it up till the desired consistency is reached.
Nutrition Info: (Per Serving): Calories- 228, Fat- 4 g, Protein- 10 g, Carbohydrates- 35 g

Blackberry Mango Crunch

Servings: 3
Cooking Time: 2 Minutes
Ingredients:
- 1 ripe banana, peeled and chopped
- 1 pear, cored and chopped
- ¼ cup whole blackberries (fresh or frozen)
- ¼ cup cashews
- 1 teaspoon maqui berry powder
- 8-9 fresh mint leaves
- 2 teaspoons freshly squeezed lemon juice
- 1 cup filtered water
- 4-5 ice cubes

Directions:
1. Combine all the ingredients in a blender jar and run it for 1 minute or until smooth and creamy.
Nutrition Info: (Per Serving): Calories- 200, Fat- 6.4 g, Protein- 3.1 g, Carbohydrates- 35 g

Oat And Walnut Berry Blast

Servings: 2
Cooking Time: 2 Minutes
Ingredients:
- ¼ cup rolled oats
- ¼ cup walnuts, chopped
- 1 cup whole blueberries (fresh or frozen)
- 2 oranges, peeled and seeded
- 1 teaspoon cinnamon powder
- 1 cup filtered water
- 3-4 ice cubes

Directions:
1. Whizz all the ingredients until well combined and serve.
Nutrition Info: (Per Serving): Calories- 218, Fat- 8 g, Protein- 6 g, Carbohydrates- 35 g

Green Chia Smoothie

Servings: 3
Cooking Time: 5 Minutes
Ingredients:
- 1 ½ cups spinach, washed and chopped
- 1 large kale leaf, chopped
- 1 cup English cucumber, chopped
- 1 small apple, cored and chopped
- 1 teaspoon freshly squeezed lemon juice
- 3 teaspoons Chia seeds, soaked
- 1 teaspoon raw organic honey
- 1 ½ cup filtered water
- 3-4 ice cubes

Directions:
1. To you blender, add the above ingredient and pulse until smooth.
Nutrition Info: (Per Serving): Calories- 100, Fat- 2.9 g, Protein- 5 g, Carbohydrates- 18.5 g

Hemp, Date And Chia Smoothie

Servings: 2
Cooking Time: 2 Minutes
Ingredients:
- 1 cup unsweetened almond milk
- ¼ teaspoon vanilla extract
- 1 dates, pitted
- 1 tablespoon hemp seeds
- ½ ripe banana, chopped
- 1 teaspoon Chia seeds, soaked
- A large handful of chopped kale
- 4-5 ice cubes

Directions:
1. Place all the ingredients into your blender and run it on medium high speed for 1-2 minutes or until done.

Nutrition Info: (Per Serving): Calories- 218, Fat- 11 g, Protein- 8 g, Carbohydrates- 31 g

Nutty Mango Green Blend

Servings: 2
Cooking Time: 5 Minutes
Ingredients:
- 1 cup fresh mango, chopped (fresh or frozen)
- 1 cup fresh baby spinach, washed and chopped
- ½ cup low fat plain yogurt
- 1 teaspoon pistachios
- 1 teaspoon peanuts
- 1 teaspoon pecan nuts
- ½ teaspoon liquid Stevia
- 2 teaspoons freshly squeezed lemon juice
- 5 ice cubes

Directions:
1. To you blender, add the above ingredient and pulse until smooth.

Nutrition Info: (Per Serving): Calories-300, Fat- 6.8 g, Protein- 12 g, Carbohydrates- 45 g

Choco- Berry Delight

Servings: 4
Cooking Time: 5 Minutes
Ingredients:
- ½ cup whole blueberries (fresh or frozen)
- ½ cup cherries, pitted
- 1 ripe banana, chopped
- 1 cup unsweetened almond milk
- 2 cups mixed greens, washed and chopped
- 1 cup baby spinach, washed and chopped
- 2 stalks celery, copped
- 2 teaspoons raw cacao powder
- 1 teapoon Chia seeds
- 3-4 ice cubes

Directions:
1. Place all the ingredients into your blender and run it on medium high speed for 1-2 minutes or until done.

Nutrition Info: (Per Serving): Calories- 310, Fat- 7.9 g, Protein- 8 g, Carbohydrates- 59 g

Coconut Blue Wonder

Servings: 2
Cooking Time: 5 Minutes
Ingredients:
- 1 cup whole blueberries (fresh or frozen)
- 1 cup organic coconut milk
- ¼ cup plain low fat yogurt
- 1 small handful of baby spinach, chopped
- 1 ½ teaspoon flaxseed powder
- 3-4 ice cubes

Directions:
1. Combine all the ingredients in a blender jar and run it for 1 minute or until smooth and creamy.

Nutrition Info: (Per Serving): Calories- 240, Fat- 11 g, Protein- 4 g, Carbohydrates- 31 g

Carrot Crunch Smoothie

Servings: 2
Cooking Time: 5 Minutes
Ingredients:
- 1 grapefruit, peeled and seeded
- 1 cup carrot, peeled and chopped
- 1 cup low fat plain yogurt
- 2 teaspoons raw, organic honey
- 3 teaspoons macadamia nuts, chopped
- 3 teaspoons almonds, chopped
- 5-6 ice cubes

Directions:
1. Place all the ingredients into the high speed blender jar and run it on high for 20 seconds until everything is well combined. Pour into serving glass and enjoy!

Nutrition Info: (Per Serving): Calories- 310, Fat- 12 g, Protein- 11 g, Carbohydrates- 39 g

Raspberry Peach Delight

Servings: 3
Cooking Time: 5 Minutes
Ingredients:
- 1 cup whole raspberries (fresh or frozen)
- 1 ½ cups peaches, pitted (fresh or frozen)
- 1 cup unsweetened, organic coconut milk

- ¼ teaspoon vanilla extract
- 2 teaspoons Chia seeds
- 2 teaspoons freshly squeezed lemon juice
- 2 teaspoons raw organic honey
- 1 cups filtered water
- 4-5 ice cubes

Directions:
1. To you blender, add the above ingredient and pulse until smooth.

Nutrition Info: (Per Serving): Calories- 161, Fat- 4.9 g, Protein- 3 g, Carbohydrates- 30 g

Super Tropi-kale Wonder

Servings: 4
Cooking Time: 5 Minutes
Ingredients:
- 1 cup pineapple, chopped
- 1 cup mango, peeled and hopped
- 2 cups mixed greens, washed and chopped
- 1 ripe banana, chopped
- 1 teaspoon Spirulina powder
- ½ teaspoon bee pollen
- 3 teaspoons Brazil nuts
- 2 teaspoons flax seeds
- 1 ½ teaspoon pure coconut oil
- 1 ¼ cup filtered water
- 3-4 ice cubes

Directions:
1. Add all the ingredients in the same order as listed above and blend until smooth and thick.

Nutrition Info: (Per Serving): Calories- 300, Fat-11 g, Protein-7.4 g, Carbohydrates-45 g

Banana-sunflower Coconut Smoothie

Servings: 2
Cooking Time: 2 Minutes
Ingredients:
- 2 ripe bananas, sliced (fresh or frozen)
- 3 teaspoons raw cacao powder
- 2 teaspoons maca powder
- 3 teaspoons coconut cream
- 2 teaspoon sunflower seeds
- 1 cup filtered water
- 1 teaspoon raw organic honey
- 4-5 ice cubes

Directions:
1. Place all the ingredients into your blender and run it on medium high speed for 1-2 minutes or until done.

Nutrition Info: (Per Serving): Calories- 200, Fat- 6.9 g, Protein- 3.6 g, Carbohydrates- 32 g

Blue And Green Wonder

Servings: 3
Cooking Time: 5 Minutes
Ingredients:
- 1 cup unsweetened almond milk
- 1 cup whole blueberries (fresh or frozen)
- 1 ripe banana, chopped
- 1 cup baby spinach, washed and chopped
- 1 cup fresh kale, stems removed and chopped
- 2 teaspoons flax seeds
- 4-5 ice cubes

Directions:
1. Add all the ingredients in the same order as listed above and blend until smooth and thick.

Nutrition Info: (Per Serving): Calories- 122, Fat- 2 g, Protein- 3 g, Carbohydrates- 25 g

Chia Flax Berry Green Smoothie

Servings: 3
Cooking Time: 5 Minutes
Ingredients:
- 1 cup unsweetened almond milk
- 2 teaspoons almond butter
- 1 cup frozen mixed berries
- 1 ripe banana, chopped
- 1 cup fresh spinach, chopped
- 2 teaspoons flaxseed powder
- 2 teaspoons Chia seeds oaked
- 1 teaspoon raw organic honey
- 4-5 ice cubes

Directions:
1. Whizz all the ingredients until well combined and serve.

Nutrition Info: (Per Serving): Calories- 360, Fat- 1.3 g, Protein- 11 g, Carbohydrates- 45 g

GREEN SMOOTHIES

The Curious Raspberry And Green Shake

Servings: 1
Cooking Time: 10 Minutes
Ingredients:
- ¼ cup raspberry
- 1 tablespoon macadamia oil
- 1 cup whole milk
- 1 pack stevia
- 1 cup spinach
- 1 cup of water

Directions:
1. Add listed ingredients to a blender
2. Blend until you get a smooth and creamy texture
3. Serve chilled and enjoy!

Nutrition Info: Calories: 292; Fat: 21g; Carbohydrates: 17g; Protein: 9g

The Coolest 5 Lettuce Green Shake

Servings: 1
Cooking Time: 10 Minutes
Ingredients:
- 1 tablespoon MCT oil
- 1 tablespoon chia seeds
- 2 cups 5 – lettuce mix salad greens
- ¾ cup whole milk yogurt
- 1 pack stevia
- 1 ½ cups of water

Directions:
1. Add listed ingredients to a blender
2. Blend until you have a smooth and creamy texture
3. Serve chilled and enjoy!

Nutrition Info: Calories: 320; Fat: 24g; Carbohydrates: 17g; Protein: 10g

Clementine Green Smoothie

Servings: 3
Cooking Time: 5 Minutes
Ingredients:
- 2-3 Clementine, peeled and deseeded
- 1 small banana, chopped
- ¼ cup fresh coconut milk
- 1 small handful of mixed greens
- A few sprigs of mint leaves
- A few fresh cilantro leaves
- ½ teaspoon raw organic honey
- 1 teaspoon freshly squeezed lemon juice
- 3-4 ice cubes

Directions:
1. Add all the ingredients into the high speed blender and whizz until smooth.

Nutrition Info: (Per Serving): Calories- 180, Fat- 3.2 g, Protein- 3.5 g, Carbohydrates- 42 g

Banana Green Smoothie

Servings: 2
Cooking Time: 10 Minutes
Ingredients:
- 2 bananas
- 1 cup strawberries
- 1 cup almond milk
- 2 cups spinach, raw
- 2 teaspoons vanilla extract

Directions:
1. Add listed ingredients to a blender
2. Blend until you have a smooth and creamy texture
3. Serve chilled and enjoy!

Nutrition Info: Calories: 212; Fat: 14.7g; Carbohydrates: 20.4g; Protein: 2.7g

Passion Green Smoothie

Servings: 2
Cooking Time: 10 Minutes
Ingredients:
- 1 cup strawberries
- 2 cups spinach, raw
- ½ cup blueberries
- ½ cup Greek yogurt
- 2 cups of water

Directions:
1. Add listed ingredients to a blender
2. Blend until you have a smooth and creamy texture
3. Serve chilled and enjoy!

Nutrition Info: Calories: 88; Fat: 1.5g; Carbohydrates: 13.9g; Protein: 6.6g

Berry Spinach Basil Smoothie

Servings: 2
Cooking Time: 5 Minutes
Ingredients:
- 1 cup unsweetened almond milk
- 1 small banana, chopped
- ½ cup blueberries (fresh or frozen)
- A small handful of baby spinach
- 6-7 fresh basil leaves
- 2 teaspoons freshly squeezed lemon juice

- 3-4 ice cubes

Directions:
1. Add all the ingredients into the high speed blender and whizz until smooth.

Nutrition Info: (Per Serving): Calories- 250, Fat- 5.8g, Protein- 5 g ,Carbohydrates- 51 g

Mango Grape Smoothie

Servings: 2
Cooking Time: 2 Minutes
Ingredients:
- ¾ cup mango, peeled and chopped
- 1 cup collard greens, stems removed and chopped
- ½ cup green grapes (seedless)
- 2 teaspoons freshly squeezed lemon juice
- A few sprigs of cilantro
- 3-4 ice cubes

Directions:
1. Just put all the ingredients into the blender and blitz until nice and smooth.

Nutrition Info: (Per Serving): Calories- 180, Fat- 1.1 g, Protein- 4 g, Carbohydrates- 45 g

Garden Variety Green And Yogurt Delight

Servings: 1
Cooking Time: 10 Minutes
Ingredients:
- 1 cup whole milk yogurt
- 1 tablespoon flaxseed, ground
- 1 cup garden greens
- 1 tablespoon MCT oil
- 1 cup of water
- 1 pack stevia

Directions:
1. Add listed ingredients to a blender
2. Blend until you have a smooth and creamy texture
3. Serve chilled and enjoy!

Nutrition Info: Calories: 334; Fat: 26g; Carbohydrates: 14g; Protein: 11g

Lovely Green Gazpacho

Servings: 2
Cooking Time: 5 Minutes
Ingredients:
- ½ cup ice
- 1 cup collard greens, chopped
- ¼ cup red bell pepper, diced
- ½ cup frozen broccoli florets
- ½ cup fresh tomatoes, chopped
- 1 garlic clove
- ¼ cup fresh cilantro, chopped
- ½ lemon, juiced
- ½ cup water

Directions:
1. Add all the ingredients except vegetables/fruits first
2. Blend until smooth
3. Add the vegetable/fruits
4. Blend until smooth
5. Add a few ice cubes and serve the smoothie
6. Enjoy!

Nutrition Info: Calories: 70; Fat: 1g; Carbohydrates: 13g; Protein: 4g

Electrifying Green Smoothie

Servings: 2
Cooking Time: 10 Minutes
Ingredients:
- ½ cup pineapple, peeled and chopped
- 2 cups almond milk
- 2 oranges, peeled
- 2 cups spinach, raw

Directions:
1. Slice the peeled oranges, then remove the seeds
2. Add listed ingredients to a blender
3. Blend until you have a smooth and creamy texture
4. Serve chilled and enjoy!

Nutrition Info: Calories: 209; Fat: 6.4g; Carbohydrates: 38.4g; Protein: 4.8g

Citrus Green Smoothie

Servings: 2
Cooking Time: 10 Minutes
Ingredients:
- 2 oranges, peeled
- 2 cups almond milk
- 1 cup strawberries
- 2 cups spinach, raw

Directions:
1. Add listed ingredients to a blender
2. Blend until you have a smooth and creamy texture
3. Serve chilled and enjoy!

Nutrition Info: Calories: 334; Fat: 28.9g; Carbohydrates: 20.8g; Protein: 4.3g

Tropical Matcha Kale

Servings: 2

Cooking Time: 5 Minutes
Ingredients:
- ½ cup ice
- 1 cup kale, chopped
- ½ cup frozen mango died
- 1 teaspoon matcha powder
- ½ cup plain kefir
- ¼ cup cold water

Directions:
1. Add all the ingredients except vegetables/fruits first
2. Blend until smooth
3. Add the vegetable/fruits
4. Blend until smooth
5. Add a few ice cubes and serve the smoothie
6. Enjoy!

Nutrition Info: Calories: 126; Fat: 2g; Carbohydrates: 23g; Protein: 6g

Greenie Genie S Moothie

Servings: 3
Cooking Time: 5 Minutes
Ingredients:
- 1 cup unsweetened almond milk
- 1 banana, chopped (fresh or frozen)
- ½ cup avocado, pitted and chopped
- 1 kiwi fruit, peeled and chopped
- 1 cup baby spinach, chopped
- 1 tablespoons raw organic honey
- A pinch of cinnamon powder
- 3-4 ice cubes

Directions:
1. Add all the ingredients into the blender and whizz until smooth.

Nutrition Info: (Per Serving): Calories- Fat- 4.5 g, Protein- 5 g, Carbohydrates- 17 g

The Wild Matcha Delight

Servings: 2
Cooking Time: 5 Minutes
Ingredients:
- 1 cup unsweetened coconut milk
- 1 teaspoon matcha powder
- ½ teaspoon cinnamon
- 1 cup baby spinach, chopped
- 1 cup wild blueberries, frozen

Directions:
1. Add all the ingredients except vegetables/fruits first
2. Blend until smooth
3. Add the vegetable/fruits
4. Blend until smooth
5. Add a few ice cubes and serve the smoothie
6. Enjoy!

Nutrition Info: Calories: 130; Fat: 3g; Carbohydrates: 21g; Protein: 5g

Dandellion Green Berry Smoothie

Servings: 2
Cooking Time: 5 Minutes
Ingredients:
- ½ cup dandelion greens, chopped
- ½ small banana, hopped
- A handful of mixed berries
- 1 cup filtered water
- 1 teaspoon coconut oil
- A pinch of cinnamon powder
- 1 teaspoon flax seed powder
- 1 teaspoon cacao powder
- 1 teaspoon raw organic honey
- ½ teaspoon Chia seeds
- ½ teaspoon hemp seeds
- 3-4 ice cubes

Directions:
1. Add all the above listed ingredients into your blender, secure the lid and blitz until smooth.

Nutrition Info: (Per Serving): Calories- 270, Fat- 16 g, Protein- 3.2 g, Carbohydrates- 35 g

A Mean Green Milk Shake

Servings: 1
Cooking Time: 10 Minutes
Ingredients:
- 1 cup whole milk
- 1 tablespoon coconut flakes, unsweetened
- 1 cup of water
- 2 cups spring mix salad
- 1 tablespoon coconut oil
- 1 pack stevia

Directions:
1. Add listed ingredients to a blender
2. Blend until you have a smooth and creamy texture
3. Serve chilled and enjoy!

Nutrition Info: Calories: 309; Fat: 23g; Carbohydrates: 18g; Protein: 9.5g

Berry Collard Green Smoothie

Servings: 3
Cooking Time: 5 Minutes
Ingredients:
- ½ avocado, pitted and chopped

- 1 small banana, chopped
- ½ cup coconut water
- ½ cup collard greens, chopped
- ½ cup pineapple, peel and chopped
- ¾ cup whole blueberries (fresh or frozen)
- 1 teaspoon freshly squeezed lemon juice
- ¼ teaspoon freshly grated ginger
- ½ teaspoon raw, organic honey
- 4-5 ice cubes

Directions:
1. Place all the ingredients in the blender and run it on high for 30 seconds or until the desired consistency is got.

Nutrition Info: (Per Serving): Calories- 166, Fat-1.8 g, Protein- 5 g, Carbohydrates- 42 g

The Deep Green Lagoon

Servings: 2
Cooking Time: 5 Minutes
Ingredients:
- ½ cup ice
- ½ cup collard greens, chopped
- 1 cup spinach, chopped
- ½ cup fresh broccoli florets, diced
- 1 pear, roughly chopped
- 1 teaspoon spirulina powder
- ½ cup of water

Directions:
1. Add all the ingredients except vegetables/fruits first
2. Blend until smooth
3. Add the vegetable/fruits
4. Blend until smooth
5. Add a few ice cubes and serve the smoothie
6. Enjoy!

Nutrition Info: Calories: 124; Fat: 1g; Carbohydrates: 30g; Protein: 4g

The Minty Cucumber

Servings: 2
Cooking Time: 5 Minutes
Ingredients:
- ½ cup ice
- 1½ cups swiss chard, chopped
- ¾ cup cucumber, diced
- 1 pear, roughly chopped
- ¼ cup fresh cilantro, chopped
- 4 fresh mint leaves, chopped
- ½ lemon, juiced
- ¼ cup water

Directions:
1. Add all the ingredients except vegetables/fruits first
2. Blend until smooth
3. Add the vegetable/fruits
4. Blend until smooth
5. Add a few ice cubes and serve the smoothie
6. Enjoy

Nutrition Info: Calories: 105; Fat: 0g; Carbohydrates: 25g; Protein: 3g

Date And Apricot Green Smoothie

Servings: 2 Large
Cooking Time: 2 Minutes
Ingredients:
- ¾ cup unsweetened almond milk
- 1 small apricot, pitted and chopped
- 1 medjool dates, pitted
- 1 small banana, chopped
- ½ cup kale, stems removed and chopped
- ½ cup baby spinach, washed
- A handful of mixed berries
- Few ice cubes

Directions:
1. Pour the ingredients into the blender and process until smooth.

Nutrition Info: (Per Serving): Calories- 202, Fat- 3.6 g, Protein- 7.6 g, Carbohydrates- 38 g

Minty Cantaloupe Smoothie

Servings: 3
Cooking Time: 5 Minutes
Ingredients:
- 1 cup cucumber, chopped
- 1 cup cantaloupe, chopped
- 2/3 cup unsweetened almond milk
- A small handful of kale, stems removed and chopped
- ½ teaspoon raw, organic honey
- ¼ vanilla extract
- 3 tablespoons fresh mint
- 3 tablespoons fresh basil
- 2 tablespoon freshly squeezed lemon juice
- 3-4 ice cubes

Directions:
1. Whizz up all the ingredients in the blender for 45 seconds and serve.

Nutrition Info: (Per Serving): Calories- 120, Fat- 1.8 g, Protein- 4.2 g, Carbohydrates- 26 g

The Green Potato Chai

Servings: 2
Cooking Time: 5 Minutes
Ingredients:
- ½ cup chilled, brewed chai
- ½ cup ice
- 1½ cups kale, chopped
- 1 pear, roughly chopped
- 1 scoop unsweetened protein powder
- ¼ teaspoon cinnamon

Directions:
1. Add all the ingredients except vegetables/fruits first
2. Blend until smooth
3. Add the vegetable/fruits
4. Blend until smooth
5. Add a few ice cubes and serve the smoothie
6. Enjoy!

Nutrition Info: Calories: 286; Fat: 1g; Carbohydrates: 43g; Protein: 29g

Cacao Mango Green Smoothie

Servings: 4
Cooking Time: 2 Minutes
Ingredients:
- 1 cup mango, peeled and chopped
- 1 cup unsweetened almond milk
- 1 cup blueberries (fresh or frozen)
- 2 cups fresh baby spinach
- 1 cup mixed greens
- 2 teaspoons Chia seeds, soaked
- 3 teaspoons raw cacao powder
- 1 teaspoon raw organic honey
- 1 teaspoon flaxseed powder
- 3-4 ice cubes

Directions:
1. Blend all the ingredients into the blender and enjoy!

Nutrition Info: (Per Serving): Calories- 339, Fat- 2.8 g, Protein- 10 g, Carbohydrates- 70 g

Blackberry Green Smoothie

Servings: 3
Cooking Time: 5 Minutes
Ingredients:
- 1 cup whole blackberries (fresh or frozen)
- 1 large apple, cored and chopped
- 2 cups fresh baby spinach
- 1 cup fresh kale, stems removed and chopped
- 1 cup fresh coconut water
- 3 teaspoons Chia seeds, soaked
- 1 teaspoon freshly squeezed lemon juice
- 3-4 ice cubes

Directions:
1. Pour the ingredients into the blender and process until smooth.

Nutrition Info: (Per Serving): Calories- 360, Fat-0.3 g, Protein- 11 g, Carbohydrates- 70 g

Tropical Apple Coconut Green Blend

Servings: 3
Cooking Time: 5 Minutes
Ingredients:
- 1 cup plain low fat yogurt
- ½ cup cucumber, deseeded and chopped
- Freshly squeezed juice of 1 lime
- 1 large green apple, cored and chopped
- ½ cup fresh coconut water
- A handful of spinach, washed and chopped
- 6-7 fresh mint leaves
- 6-7 ice cubes
- 1 teaspoon raw organic honey (optional)

Directions:
1. Pour the ingredients into the blender and process until smooth.

Nutrition Info: (Per Serving): Calories- 158, Fat- 0.3 g, Protein- 12 g, Carbohydrates- 30 g

Lemon Cilantro Delight

Servings: 2
Cooking Time: 5 Minutes
Ingredients:
- ½ cup ice
- 1 cup dandelion greens, chopped
- 2 celery stalks, roughly chopped
- 1 pear, roughly chopped
- 1 tablespoon chia seeds
- ¼ cup fresh cilantro, chopped
- Juice of ½ lemon
- ¼ cup water

Directions:
1. Add all the ingredients except vegetables/fruits first
2. Blend until smooth
3. Add the vegetable/fruits
4. Blend until smooth
5. Add a few ice cubes and serve the smoothie
6. Enjoy!

Nutrition Info: Calories: 200; Fat: 5g; Carbohydrates: 34g; Protein: 5g

Cilantro And Citrus Glass

Servings: 2
Cooking Time: 5 Minutes
Ingredients:
- ½ cup ice
- 2 cups arugula
- ½ cup celery, diced
- 1 grapefruit, peeled and segmented
- 1 handful fresh cilantro leaves, chopped
- ½ lemon, juiced
- ½ cup water

Directions:
1. Add all the ingredients except vegetables/fruits first
2. Blend until smooth
3. Add the vegetable/fruits
4. Blend until smooth
5. Add a few ice cubes and serve the smoothie
6. Enjoy!

Nutrition Info: Calories: 75; Fat: 1g; Carbohydrates: 16g; Protein: 3g

Cherry Acai Berry Smoothie

Servings: 2
Cooking Time: 2 Minutes
Ingredients:
- 1 cup whole Acai berries (fresh or frozen)
- 1 large banana, sliced (fresh or frozen)
- 1 cup fresh cherries, pitted
- ½ cup filtered water or coconut water
- A large handful of minced greens
- 2-3 ice cubes

Directions:
1. Place all the ingredients in the blender and run it on high for 30 seconds or until the desired consistency is got.

Nutrition Info: (Per Serving): Calories- 360, Fat- 6.8 g, Protein- 6 g, Carbohydrates- 75 g

Pineapple And Cucumber Cooler

Servings: 3-4
Cooking Time: 5 Minutes
Ingredients:
- 1 green apple, cored and chopped
- 1 cup pineapple, peeled and chopped
- 1 green cucumber, deseeded and chopped
- 5-6 celery stalks, chopped
- A handful of kale leaves, stems removed and chopped
- 1/3 cup fresh parsley
- 1 teaspoon freshly grated ginger
- 1 tablespoon freshly squeezed lemon juice
- 3-4 ice cubes

Directions:
1. Add all the ingredients into the blender jar and pulse it on high for 30 seconds or until smooth.

Nutrition Info: (Per Serving): Calories-226, Fat- 1.8 g, Protein- 7.8 g, Carbohydrates- 36 g

Coco-banann Green Smoothie

Servings: 3
Cooking Time: 5 Minutes
Ingredients:
- 1 cup fresh kale, stems removed and chopped
- 1 cup baby spinach, washed
- 1 ½ cups pineapple, peeled and chopped
- ½ cup fresh coconut milk
- 1 large ripe banana, chopped
- 2 tablespoons freshly squeezed lime juice
- 1 tablespoon fresh parsley
- 3-4 ice cubes

Directions:
1. To make this smoothie, place everything into the blender and pulse until smooth. Serve immediately.

Nutrition Info: (Per Serving): Calories 250, Fat 12.7 g, Protein- 4.7 g, Carbohydrates- 35 g

VEGAN AND VEGETARIAN DIET SMOOTHIES

Lime & Green Tea Smoothie Bowl

Servings: 2
Cooking Time: 10 Min
Ingredients:
- 1/2 cup coconut juice/ water
- 1 cup fresh spinach leaves
- 1 large frozen banana slices
- 1/4 cup avocado slices
- 2 tsp lime zest
- 1 tbsp. and 1 tsp lime juice
- 3 ice cubes
- 2 tsp maple syrup
- 1/2 tsp good quality Matcha Green Tea powder
- Toppings:
- Granola, chopped into pieces
- Coconut flakes
- Coconut cream

Directions:
1. Put all the ingredients in a high-speed blender, except the toppings. Blend until smooth.
2. Transfer in glasses or bowls. Put toppings as much as you want. Enjoy!

Nutrition Info: (Per Serving): Cal 437 Total Fat 22.4 g, Carbs 55.4 g, Fiber 10.9 g, Protein 10.4 g, Sodium 44 mg Sugars 31.9 g

Super Avocado Smoothie

Servings: 2
Cooking Time: 5 Min
Ingredients:
- 1 medium avocado
- 1 cup blueberries
- 1 cup frozen strawberries
- ½ cup frozen raspberries
- ¼ cup reduced fat vanilla yogurt
- 1 cup orange juice
- ½ cup filtered water
- 1 tablespoon maple syrup
- 15 mint leaves

Directions:
1. Peel and pit avocado and add to a blender.
2. Add blueberries, strawberries, raspberries, yogurt, orange juice, water, maple syrup and mint.
3. Pulse for 1 minute until smooth and serve immediately.

Nutrition Info: (Per Serving):156 Cal, 8 g total fat (1 g sat. fat), 0 mg chol., 64 mg sodium, 54 g carb., 8g fiber, 3 g protein.

Avocado And Blueberry Smoothie

Servings: 2
Cooking Time: 10 Min
Ingredients:
- 1 cup orange juice
- 1/2 cup mineral water
- 1 haas avocado, seeded and peeled
- 1 cup fresh blueberries
- 1/4 cup vegan yogurt
- 1 tbsp. maple syrup
- 1 cup frozen blueberries
- 1/2 cup frozen raspberries
- 1/4 cup fresh mint leaves
- Pinch of Celtic salt

Directions:
1. Throw everything in a high speed blender. Process until smooth.
2. Serve right away.

Nutrition Info: (Per Serving): Cal 111 Total Fat 12.3 g, Carbs 39.2 g, Fiber 8.1 g, Protein 11 g, Sodium 206 mg Sugars 29 g

Chia, Blueberry & Banana Smoothie

Servings: 2
Cooking Time: 5 Min
Ingredients:
- 2 medium fresh bananas
- 1 cup frozen blueberries
- 1 cup fat free milk, unsweetened
- 2 tablespoons Chia Seeds
- 1 cup ice cubes

Directions:
1. Peel banana, chop roughly and place in a blender along with blueberries, milk, chia seeds and ice.
2. Pulse 1 minute until smooth and serve immediately.

Nutrition Info: (Per Serving):220 Cal, 1.5 g total fat (0.5 g sat. fat), 0 mg chol., 71 mg sodium, 48 g carb., 3.4g fiber, 5.5 g protein.

Spinach, Grape, & Coconut Smoothie

Servings: 2
Cooking Time: 5 Min
Ingredients:
- 2 cups seedless green grapes
- 2 cups baby spinach
- ½ cup reduced fat coconut milk
- 1 cup ice cubes

Directions:

1. In a blender, place grapes, spinach and ice, and pour in milk.
2. Pulse for 1 minute until smooth and serve immediately.
Nutrition Info: (Per Serving):194 Cal, 2 g total fat (0 g sat. fat), 0 mg chol., 108 mg sodium, 31 g carb., 4g fiber, 0 g protein.

Mango, Lime & Spinach Smoothie

Servings: 2
Cooking Time: 5 Min
Ingredients:
- 1 cup seedless green grapes
- 2 cups baby spinach
- 1 large Mango
- 2 tablespoons lime juice
- 1 cup ice cubes

Directions:
1. Peel and core mango, roughly chop flesh and place in a blender.
2. Add grapes, spinach, lime juice, ice and pulse for 1 minute until smooth.
3. Serve immediately.
Nutrition Info: (Per Serving):167 Cal, 0 g total fat (0 g sat. fat), 0 mg chol., 67 mg sodium, 64 g carb., 5g fiber, 6 g protein.

Beet And Grapefruit Smoothie

Servings: 1
Cooking Time: 5 Min
Ingredients:
- 1/2 Cucumber, peeled and diced
- 1/2 small red beet, peeled and diced
- 1 apple, cored and chopped
- 6 tbsps. Grapefruit juice
- 4 ice cubes

Directions:
1. In a high speed blender, add cucumber and blend until it breaks into pieces. Add apple, beet and blend until smooth.
2. Add water if it's too hard to blend. Push the sides and blend again until you reach fine consistency. Add ice, grapefruit juice and blend.
3. Serve right away.
Nutrition Info: (Per Serving): Cal 208 Total Fat 1.2 g, Carbs 45.9 g, Fiber 4 g, Protein 6 g, Sodium 33 mg Sugars 25 g

Healthy Kiwi Smoothie

Servings: 2
Cooking Time: 20 Min

Ingredients:
- 1 celery stalk
- 2 medium granny smith apples, cored
- 1 kiwi fruit, peeled and chopped
- 1/3 cup parsley leaves
- 1 tbsp. grated ginger
- Maple syrup
- 2 tsp lime juice

Directions:
1. Add all ingredients in a blender, except lime juice and blend until smooth. Taste and adjust sweetness with maple syrup.
2. Stir in lime juice and serve.
Nutrition Info: (Per Serving): Cal 82 Total Fat 1 g, Carbs 20 g, Fiber 0 g, Protein 1 g, Sodium 9 mg Sugars 18 g

Green Smoothie

Servings: 2
Cooking Time: 5 Min
Ingredients:
- 2 medium green apples
- Half of a medium avocado
- 1-inch ginger piece
- 1 cup baby spinach
- 1 cup coconut water
- 1 tablespoon flax oil
- 1 cup ice cubes

Directions:
1. Peel apple, core, slice and place in a blender. Peel and pit avocado and add to blender.
2. Peel and dice ginger and add to blender along with spinach, coconut water, flax oil and ice cubes.
3. Pulse for 1 minute until smooth and creamy and then serve over ice.
Nutrition Info: (Per Serving):156 Cal, 1 g total fat (0.2 g sat. fat), 0 mg chol., 54 mg sodium, 38 g carb., 6.5g fiber, 3.6 g protein.

Pina Colada Smoothie

Servings: 2
Cooking Time: 5 Min
Ingredients:
- 1 cup pineapple chunks
- 1 banana
- 2 teaspoons honey
- 1 cup reduced fat coconut milk, unsweetened
- ½ cup ice cubes
- 2 Pineapple wedges, for garnish

Directions:

1. Peel banana, chop roughly and place in a blender along with pineapple, honey, coconut milk and ice cubes.
2. Pulse for 1 minute until smooth and divide smoothie between two serving glasses.
3. Garnish each serving glass with a pineapple wedge and serve immediately.

Nutrition Info: (Per Serving):158 Cal, 6.6 g total fat (2 g sat. fat), 0 mg chol., 39 mg sodium, 23 g carb., 2g fiber, 2.7 g protein.

Apple, Carrot, Ginger & Fennel Smoothie

Servings: 2
Cooking Time: 5 Min
Ingredients:
- 1 medium apple
- 2 medium carrots
- 2 tablespoons peeled ginger slices
- 1 cup sliced fennel bulb
- 1 tablespoon honey
- 1 cup apple juice
- 1 tablespoons lemon juice
- 1 cup ice cubes

Directions:
1. Peel and core apple, cut into slices and place in a blender.
2. Peel carrots, dice and add to blender along with ginger, fennel bulb, honey, apple juice, lemon juice and ice cubes.
3. Pulse for 1 minute until smoothie and serve immediately.

Nutrition Info: (Per Serving):144 Cal, 0 g total fat (0 g sat. fat), 0 mg chol., 63 mg sodium, 36 g carb., 5g fiber, 2 g protein.

Strawberry Watermelon Smoothie

Servings: 2
Cooking Time: 5 Min
Ingredients:
- 1 1/2 cups sliced watermelons, seeds removed
- 1 cup frozen strawberries
- 1/2 frozen ripe banana, sliced
- 1/2 cup unsweetened almond milk
- 1 lime juice
- 1 tbsp. chia seeds

Directions:
1. Add all ingredients in a blender. Process until smooth and fine texture. Adjust sweetness with more banana.
2. Top with more chia seeds.

Nutrition Info: (Per Serving): Cal 182 Total Fat 6.2 g, Carbs 30 g, Fiber 9 g, Protein 5 g, Sodium 48 mg Sugars 14 g

Caramel Banana Smoothie

Servings: 2
Cooking Time: 10 Min
Ingredients:
- 1 1/2 cups almond milk
- 3 Medjool dates, pitted
- 2 medium frozen bananas, sliced
- 1 scoop of Vegan Vanilla Ice Cream
- 1 tbsp. almond butter

Directions:
1. Add everything in a blender and blend until smooth.
2. Garnish with some shaved chocolate on top or serve as is.

Nutrition Info: (Per Serving): Cal 140 Total Fat 7 g, Carbs 13 g, Fiber 2 g, Protein 7 g, Sodium 330 mg Sugars 60 g

Raspberry Smoothie

Servings: 2
Cooking Time: 5 Min
Ingredients:
- 1 cup water
- 1 cup frozen raspberries
- 1 large sliced frozen bananas
- 2 tbsps. Lime juice
- 1 tsp coconut oil
- 1 tsp agave syrup

Directions:
1. In a high-speed blender, add all ingredients and process until smooth.
2. You can add ice if you want or add more frozen bananas. Adjust taste with agave syrup.

Nutrition Info: (Per Serving): Cal 480 Total Fat 1 g, Carbs 126 g, Fiber 9 g, Protein 2 g, Sodium 20 mg Sugars 28 g

Chai Tea Smoothie

Servings: 2
Cooking Time: 10 Min
Ingredients:
- 1 cup unsweetened almond milk
- 1 cup coconut juice
- 1/4 cup chopped dates, soaked
- 1 tsp vanilla extract
- 1/2 tsp cinnamon powder

- 1/4 tsp ginger powder
- 1/8 tsp nutmeg powder
- 1/8 tsp cardamom powder
- Pinch of cloves powder
- Pinch of Himalayan sea salt
- 2 large frozen bananas, sliced
- 1 cup crushed ice
- 1 tbsp. chia seeds

Directions:
1. Add everything in a high-speed blender. Blend until smooth and creamy.
2. Serve right away!

Nutrition Info: (Per Serving): Cal 227 Total Fat 1 g, Carbs 52 g, Fiber 6 g, Protein 3 g, Sodium 280 mg Sugars 35 g

Chard, Lime & Mint Smoothies

Servings: 2
Cooking Time: 5 Min
Ingredients:
- 5 ½ ounces honeydew melon
- 3 ounces kiwifruit
- 2 cups green Swiss chards
- ½ cup soda, lime-flavored
- ¼ cup chopped mint
- 3 tablespoons reduced fat vanilla milk
- ⅛ Teaspoon salt
- 3 tablespoons lime juice
- 1 cup ice cubes

Directions:
1. Peel and core melon, cut into cubes and place in a blender.
2. Peel and core kiwifruit and add to melon along with soda, mint and milk.
3. Remove stems of chards, discard, discard leaves into strips and add to blender.
4. Add ice and pulse for 1 minute until smooth. Add more lime juice if smoothie is thick.
5. Serve immediately.

Nutrition Info: (Per Serving):67 Cal, 0.7 g total fat (0 g sat. fat), 0 mg chol., 267 mg sodium, 16 g carb., 3g fiber, 2 g protein.

Mango Smoothie

Servings: 2
Cooking Time: 5 Min
Ingredients:
- 1 1/2 cups orange juice
- 1/2 cup water
- 1/4 cup sliced avocado
- 1/2 tsp lime zest, grated
- 2 cups frozen sweet mango
- 1 tsp maple syrup

Directions:
1. Place all the ingredients in a blender. Blend until smooth and fine texture. Add more water if too thick and blend again.
2. To adjust sweetness, add more maple syrup. Enjoy while still cold!

Nutrition Info: (Per Serving): Cal 270 Total Fat 1.5 g, Carbs 53 g, Fiber 6 g, Protein 16 g, Sodium 0 mg Sugars 37 g

BRAIN HEALTH SMOOTHIES

The Gritty Coffee Shake

Servings: 1
Cooking Time: 10 Minutes
Ingredients:
- 2 cups strongly brewed coffee, chilled
- 1-ounce Macadamia Nuts
- 1 tablespoon chia seeds
- 1 tablespoon MCT oil
- 1-2 packets Stevia, optional

Directions:
1. Add all the listed ingredients to a blender
2. Blend on high until smooth and creamy
3. Enjoy your smoothie!

Nutrition Info: Calories: 395; Fat: 39g; Carbohydrates: 11g; Protein: 5.2g

Grapefruit Spinach Smoothie

Servings: 2
Cooking Time: 10 Minutes
Ingredients:
- 2 bananas green, peeled and frozen
- 4 cups spinach, fresh or frozen
- 1 cup green tea, strongly brewed
- 2 grapefruits, peeled and frozen
- 2 cups pineapple, chopped and frozen
- ½ cup full-fat coconut milk, canned
- 4 tablespoons whey protein isolate
- 10 ice cubes

Directions:
1. Add all the listed ingredients to a blender
2. Blend until you have a smooth and creamy texture
3. Serve chilled and enjoy!

Nutrition Info: Calories: 164; Fat: 1.4g; Carbohydrates: 36g; Protein: 4.1g

Mango- Chia- Coconut Smoothie

Servings: 3
Cooking Time: 5 Minutes
Ingredients:
- 2 cups unsweetened organic coconut milk
- 1 cup mixed berries (fresh or frozen)
- 1 cup mango, chopped (fresh or frozen)
- 1 cup fresh kale, stems removed and chopped
- 1 large banana, chopped (fresh or frozen)
- 2 tablespoons Chia seeds, soaked
- 3 teaspoons of cashew butter
- ¼ cup of filtered water

Directions:
1. Add all the ingredients into the blender jar one by one, secure the lid firmly and whizz for 30 seconds or until done.

Nutrition Info: (Per Serving): Calories- 170, Fat- 6.8 g, Protein- 5 g, Carbohydrates- 25 g

Pear 'n' Kale Smoothie

Servings: 2-3
Cooking Time: 5 Minutes
Ingredients:
- 1 large pear, peeled, cored and chopped
- 1 green apple, peeled, cored and chopped
- ½ cup pineapple, peeled and chipped
- 1 cup fresh kale, stems removed and chopped
- 1 cup mixed greens, washed and chopped
- 1 tablespoon freshly squeezed lemon juice
- 4 ounces of filtered water

Directions:
1. Combine all the ingredients in the blender and whip it on high for 30 seconds till the smoothie is thick and well combined.

Nutrition Info: (Per Serving): Calories- 250, Fat- 1.2 g, Protein- 3.2 g, Carbohydrates- 64 g

Apple-papaya Medley

Servings: 2-3
Cooking Time: 5 Minutes
Ingredients:
- ¾ cup unsweetened almond milk
- 1 cup papaya, chopped
- 1 small banana, chopped 9fresh of frozen)
- 1 large apple, cored and chopped
- 1 cup fresh kale, stems removed
- 1 cup baby spinach
- 1 teaspoon raw organic honey
- 1 tablespoon freshly squeezed lemon juice
- 3-4 ice cubes

Directions:
1. Blend all the ingredients in your high speed blender fir 20 seconds and serve immediately.

Nutrition Info: (Per Serving): Calories- 197, Fat- 3.2 g, Protein- 4 g, Carbohydrates- 35 g

Rosemary And Lemon Garden Smoothie

Servings: 1
Cooking Time: 10 Minutes
Ingredients:
- 1 stalk fresh rosemary
- 1 tablespoon lemon juice, fresh

- ½ cup whole milk yogurt
- 1 cup garden greens
- 1 tablespoon pepitas
- 1 tablespoon olive oil
- 1 tablespoon flaxseed, ground
- 1 pack stevia
- 1 ½ cups of water

Directions:
1. Add listed ingredients to a blender
2. Blend until you get a smooth and creamy texture
3. Serve chilled and enjoy!

Nutrition Info: Calories: 312; Fat: 25g; Carbohydrates: 14g; Protein: 9g

Orange- Broccoli Green Monster

Servings: 2
Cooking Time: 5 Minutes
Ingredients:
- ½ cup chopped carrot
- ½ cup freshly squeezed orange juice
- A large handful of fresh kale, stems removed
- 1 large apple, cored and chopped
- 1 cup tightly packed baby spinach
- 1 banana, chopped (fresh or frozen)
- 1 handful of broccoli florets
- 1 tablespoon freshly squeeze lemon juice

Directions:
1. Load your blender jar with all the ingredients listed above and whizz until smooth and frothy.

Nutrition Info: (Per Serving): Calories- 255, Fat- 1.5 g, Protein- 5.2 g, Carbohydrates- 65 g

A Whole Melon Surprise

Servings: 2
Cooking Time: 5 Minutes
Ingredients:
- 1 tablespoon chia seeds
- 4 ice cubes
- 1 fresh banana
- 1 cup cantaloupe
- 1 cup honeydew
- 1 cup plain coconut yogurt
- 1 cup unsweetened coconut milk

Directions:
1. Add all the ingredients except vegetables/fruits first
2. Blend until smooth
3. Add the vegetable/fruits
4. Blend until smooth
5. Add a few ice cubes and serve the smoothie
6. Enjoy!

Nutrition Info: Calories: 134; Fat: 2g; Carbohydrates: 29g; Protein: 3g

Berry Berry Smoothie

Servings: 4
Cooking Time: 10 Minutes
Ingredients:
- 2 bananas
- 3 cups blueberries, frozen
- 2 cups almond milk
- 2 tablespoons almond butter
- 2 handfuls ice

Directions:
1. Add all the listed ingredients to a blender
2. Blend until you have a smooth and creamy texture
3. Serve chilled and enjoy!

Nutrition Info: Calories: 352; Fat: 27g; Carbohydrates: 41.5g; Protein: 4.7g

Matcha Coconut Smoothie

Servings: 2
Cooking Time: 5 Minutes
Ingredients:
- 3 tablespoons white beans
- ½ teaspoon matcha green tea powder
- 1 whole banana, cubed
- 1 cup of frozen mango, chunked
- 2 kale leaves, torn
- 2 tablespoon coconut, shredded
- 1 cup of water

Directions:
1. Add all the listed ingredients to a blender
2. Blend on high until you have a smooth and creamy texture
3. Serve chilled and enjoy!

Nutrition Info: Calories: 291; Fat: 25g; Carbohydrates: 18g; Protein: 5g

Bright Rainbow Health

Servings: 2
Cooking Time: 5 Minutes
Ingredients:
- 1 tablespoon hemp seeds
- ¼ cup pomegranate arils
- 1 cup plain low-fat Greek yogurt
- 1 cup frozen tropical fruit mix
- 1 cup frozen strawberries
- 1 cup unsweetened vanilla almond milk

Directions:

1. Add all the ingredients except vegetables/fruits first
2. Blend until smooth
3. Add the vegetable/fruits
4. Blend until smooth
5. Add a few ice cubes and serve the smoothie
6. Enjoy!

Nutrition Info: Calories: 438; Fat: 11g; Carbohydrates: 91g; Protein: 7g

Berry- Green Tea Fusion Smoothie

Servings: 2
Cooking Time: 15 Minutes
Ingredients:
- 1/3 cup filtered water
- 1 green tea bag
- 1 cup blueberries (fresh or frozen)
- 1 small banana, chopped (fresh or frozen)
- ½ cup raspberries (fresh or frozen)
- 6 ounces of low fat, plain soy milk
- 1/3 teaspoon of vanilla extract
- 5-6 cubes of ice

Directions:
1. Boil the water in a small vessel o microwave it till it nearing the boiling point.
2. Then place the tea bag into the hot water and let it steep for about 10 minutes or until the green tea is nicely infused.
3. Allow the tea to cool down to room temperature.
4. Once cooled, add the tea and the remaining ingredients into the blend and process until smooth.
5. Pour into serving glasses and serve immediately.

Nutrition Info: (Per Serving): Calories- 120, Fat- 1.4 g, Protein- 1.8 g, Carbohydrates- 30 g

Mixed- Berry Wonder

Servings: 2
Cooking Time: 2 Minutes
Ingredients:
- 1 ½ cups mixed berries of your choice (fresh or frozen)
- 1 cup unsweetened almond mil
- 1 small banana, chopped (fresh or frozen)
- 2 teaspoons flaxseed powder
- ½ teaspoon raw organic honey
- 4-5 ice cubes

Directions:
1. Place all the ingredients into your blender jar and whip it up on high until the smoothie is nice and thick. Enjoy immediately.

Nutrition Info: (Per Serving): Calories- 262, Fat- 4.1 g, Protein- 11 g, Carbohydrates- 49 g

Tropical Greens Smoothie

Servings: 2
Cooking Time: 10 Minutes
Ingredients:
- 2 cups mango chunks, frozen
- 3 coconut powder, unsweetened
- 2 cups leafy greens
- ½ cup lime juice
- 2 cups leafy greens
- 2 cups pineapple chunk, frozen

Directions:
1. Add all the listed ingredients to a blender
2. Blend until you have a smooth and creamy texture
3. Serve chilled and enjoy!

Nutrition Info: Calories: 224; Fat: 1.2g; Carbohydrates: 54.2g; Protein: 3.2g

Hale 'n' Kale Banana Smoothie

Servings: 1
Cooking Time: 2 Minutes
Ingredients:
- 1 cup fresh kale, chopped (stems removed)
- 1 handful blueberries (fresh or frozen)
- 1 small banana, chopped (fresh or frozen)
- ½ teaspoon Chia seeds
- ½ cup filtered water

Directions:
1. Add the kale, berries, banana, Chia seeds and water into your blender jar and process on high for 20 seconds or until smooth and frothy.

Nutrition Info: (Per Serving): Calories- 201, Fat- 1.2 g, Protein- 3.9 g, Carbohydrates- 44 g

The Blueberry Bliss

Servings: 1
Cooking Time: 10 Minutes
Ingredients:
- ¼ cup frozen blueberries, unsweetened
- 16 ounces unsweetened almond milk, vanilla
- 4 ounces heavy cream
- 1 scoop vanilla whey protein
- 1 pack stevia

Directions:
1. Add listed ingredients to a blender
2. Blend until you have a smooth and creamy texture
3. Serve chilled and enjoy!

Nutrition Info: Calories: 302; Fat: 25g; Carbohydrates: 4g; Protein: 15g

Nutty Bean "n"berry Smoothie

Servings: 2-3
Cooking Time: 5 Minutes
Ingredients:
- 1 cup blueberries (fresh or frozen)
- 1 cup whole strawberries (fresh or frozen)
- 1 large, raw brazil nut (roughly chopped)
- ½ cup cannellini beans (soaked overnight, drained and rinsed)
- 2 teaspoons sunflower seeds
- 2 teaspoon flax seed powder
- 1 ½ cups of filtered water

Directions:
1. Load your high speed blender jar with all the ingredients and puree until thick and smooth.

Nutrition Info: (Per Serving): Calories- 163, Fat- 6.4 g, Protein- 6.3 g, Carbohydrates- 23 g

The Wisest Watermelon Glass

Servings: 2
Cooking Time: 5 Minutes
Ingredients:
- 1 tablespoon chia seeds
- 1 cup plain coconut yogurt
- 1 cup frozen cauliflower, riced
- 1 cup frozen strawberries
- 1 cup coconut milk, unsweetened
- 1½ cups watermelon, chopped

Directions:
1. Add all the ingredients except vegetables/fruits first
2. Blend until smooth
3. Add the vegetable/fruits
4. Blend until smooth
5. Add a few ice cubes and serve the smoothie
6. Enjoy!

Nutrition Info: Calories: 130; Fat: 2g; Carbohydrates: 22g; Protein: 8g

Berry Infusion Smoothie

Servings: 2
Cooking Time: 2 Minutes
Ingredients:
- ½ cup freshly prepared pomegranate juice
- ½ large banana, chopped (fresh or frozen)
- ½ cup blueberries (fresh or frozen)
- ½ cup raspberries (fresh or frozen)
- A handful of pineapple chunks
- 2 tablespoons Chia seeds, soaked
- A few ice cubes

Directions:
1. Add all the ingredients into your blender jar, secure the lid firmly and whizz for 30 seconds or until the smoothie is thick and creamy.

Nutrition Info: (Per Serving): Calories- 378, Fat- 4.5 g, Protein- 25 g, Carbohydrates- 68 g

Mang0-soy Smoothie

Servings: 1-2
Cooking Time: 5 Minutes
Ingredients:
- 1 cup mango, chopped
- 1 cup low fat soy milk
- A handful of fresh spinach, washed and chopped
- 2 tablespoons avocado flesh
- ½ teaspoon vanilla extract
- 2 tablespoons raw organic honey or agave nectar
- 4-5 ice cubes

Directions:
1. In a blender, combine all the above listed ingredients and blend until nice and smooth.

Nutrition Info: (Per Serving): Calories- 301, Fat- 7.7 g, Protein- 8.2 g, Carbohydrates- 59 g

Pomegranate, Tangerine And Ginger Smoothie

Servings: 2
Cooking Time: 5 Minutes
Ingredients:
- ½ cup pomegranate
- 1-inch ginger root, crushed
- 1 cup tangerine
- A pinch of Himalayan pink salt

Directions:
1. Toss the pomegranate, ginger roots and tangerine into your blender
2. Add a pinch of Himalayan salt
3. Serve chilled and enjoy!

Nutrition Info: Calories: 121; Fat: 6g; Carbohydrates: 20g; Protein: 4g

Great Nutty Lion

Servings: 2
Cooking Time: 5 Minutes
Ingredients:
- 1 tablespoon almond butter

- 1 tablespoon chia seeds
- 4 ice cubes
- ¾ cup plain low-fat Greek yogurt
- 1 cup baby spinach
- 1 cup unsweetened almond milk
- 2 fresh bananas

Directions:
1. Add all the ingredients except vegetables/fruits first
2. Blend until smooth
3. Add the vegetable/fruits
4. Blend until smooth
5. Add a few ice cubes and serve the smoothie
6. Enjoy!

Nutrition Info: Calories: 250; Fat: 10g; Carbohydrates: 51g; Protein: 8g

Sweet Pea Smoothie

Servings: 2
Cooking Time: 10 Minutes
Ingredients:
- 2 cups sweet peas
- 1 cup blueberries
- 1 teaspoon honey
- 2 bananas
- 2 cups almond milk
- 2 tablespoons chia seeds

Directions:
1. Add all the listed ingredients to a blender
2. Blend until you have a smooth and creamy texture
3. Serve chilled and enjoy!

Nutrition Info: Calories: 202; Fat: 4.1g; Carbohydrates: 38.4g; Protein: 6.8g

Cacao-goji Berry Marvel

Servings: 2 Small
Cooking Time: 5 Minutes
Ingredients:
- 1 cup unsweetened almond milk
- 1 large banana, chopped (preferably frozen)
- ¼ cup Goji berries
- 3-4 fresh kale leaves, stems removed
- 1 ½ teaspoon cacao powder
- 3 teaspoon almond butter
- ¼ teaspoon cinnamon powder
- 4-6 ice cubes

Directions:
1. Load your blender with all the smoothie ingredients and process it on medium speed until the smoothie is ready. Serve immediately.

Nutrition Info: (Per Serving): Calories- 345, Fat- 10 g, Protein- 12 g, Carbohydrates- 57 g

Cheery Charlie Checker

Servings: 2
Cooking Time: 5 Minutes
Ingredients:
- 1 cup skim milk
- 1 cup frozen blueberries
- 1 fresh banana
- ¾ cup plain low-fat Greek yogurt
- ½ cup frozen cherries
- ½ cup frozen strawberries
- 1 tablespoon chia seeds

Directions:
1. Add all the ingredients except vegetables/fruits first
2. Blend until smooth
3. Add the vegetable/fruits
4. Blend until smooth
5. Add a few ice cubes and serve the smoothie
6. Enjoy!

Nutrition Info: Calories: 162; Fat: 1g; Carbohydrates: 33g; Protein: 8g

Cucumber Kiwi Crush

Servings: 2
Cooking Time: 5 Minutes
Ingredients:
- 1 cup green cucumber, roughly chopped
- 1 large kiwi, peeled and chopped
- ½ cp plain low fat yogurt
- ½ cup freshly prepared tangerine juice
- 1 cup fresh baby spinach, washed and chopped
- ½ avocado, peeled and chopped
- 1 teaspoon of freshly squeezed lemon juice
- A small handful of mint leaves
- A handful of ice cubes

Directions:
1. Combine all the ingredients in the blender and process until there are no lumps. Serve immediately.

Nutrition Info: (Per Serving): Calories-185, Fat- 7.8 g, Protein- 5.2 g, Carbohydrates- 32 g

3 Spice-almond Smoothie

Servings: 1 Large
Cooking Time: 5 Minutes
Ingredients:
- ¾ cup unsweetened almond milk
- 1 banana, sliced (fresh or frozen)

- A handful of fresh kale, stems removed
- 1 teaspoon almond butter
- A pinch of nutmeg powder
- 1 pinch of cinnamon powder
- ¼ teaspoon of freshly grated ginger
- ½ teaspoon of raw organic honey

Directions:
1. Place all the ingredients into the high speed blender jar and run it on high for 20 seconds until everything is well combined. Pour into serving glass and enjoy!

Nutrition Info: (Per Serving): Calories- 238, Fat- 10 g, Protein- 5.5 g, Carbohydrates- 39 g

Brain Nutrition-analyzer

Servings: 2
Cooking Time: 5 Minutes
Ingredients:
- 4 large ice cubes
- ¾ cup plain-low-fat Greek yogurt
- 1 cup baby spinach
- 1 cup unsweetened vanilla almond milk
- 2 fresh bananas
- 1 tablespoon almond butter
- 1 tablespoon peanut butter

Directions:
1. Add all the ingredients except vegetables/fruits first
2. Blend until smooth
3. Add the vegetable/fruits
4. Blend until smooth
5. Add a few ice cubes and serve the smoothie
6. Enjoy!

Nutrition Info: Calories: 147; Fat: 7g; Carbohydrates: 21g; Protein: 4g

Cinnammon-apple Green Smoothie

Servings: 2
Cooking Time: 5 Minutes
Ingredients:
- ¾ cup unsweetened almond milk
- 1 cup fresh kale, stems removed
- 1 cup baby spinach, washed and chopped
- 1 large apple, peeled, cored and chopped
- 1 large banana, chopped (fresh or frozen)
- 1 teaspoon raw, organic honey
- ½ teaspoon cinnamon powder
- 3-4 ice cubes

Directions:
1. To your blender jar, add all the above mentioned ingredients and process until smooth.

Nutrition Info: (Per Serving): Calories-243, Fat- 3.2 g, Protein- 4.5 g, Carbohydrates- 47 g

Apple- Blueberry Smoothie

Servings: 2
Cooking Time: 5 Minutes
Ingredients:
- 1 cup freshly prepared apple juice
- 1 cup blueberries (fresh or frozen)
- ½ cup raspberries (fresh or frozen)
- ¼ cup Goji berries (fresh or frozen)
- 1 small banana, chopped (fresh or frozen)
- 3 teaspoons hemp seed powder
- 1 teaspoon Chia seeds, soaked
- 1 teaspoon Acai powder
- ½ tablespoon organic coconut oil

Directions:
1. Load the blender jar with above listed items and blend until smooth and thick. Serve immediately.

Nutrition Info: (Per Serving): Calories- 399, Fat- 12.9 g, Protein- 6.9 g, Carbohydrates- 70 g

BEAUTY SMOOTHIES

Berry Dessert Smoothie

Servings: 2
Cooking Time: 5 Minutes
Ingredients:
- ¼ cup unsweetened almond milk
- 1 cup low fat plain yogurt
- 1 cup strawberries (fresh or frozen)
- 1 cup blueberries (fresh or frozen)
- 1 large banana, chopped (fresh or frozen)
- 1 teaspoon freshly squeezed lemon juice
- ¼ teaspoon cinnamon powder
- 3-4 ice cubes

Directions:
1. Place all the above ingredients into the blender jar and process until the mixture is thick and creamy.

Nutrition Info: (Per Serving): Calories- 265, Fat- 3.8 g, Protein- 10 g, Carbohydrates- 50 g

Min-tea Mango Rejuvinating Smoothie

Servings: 2
Cooking Time: 5 Minutes
Ingredients:
- ½ cup freshly brewed green tea (1/2 cup water+ 1 tea bag)
- ½ cup baby spinach, washed and chopped
- ½ cup mangos, cooped
- 1 teaspoon pure coconut oil
- 4-5 fresh mint leaves
- A tiny pinch of sea salt
- 1 teaspoon of freshly squeezed lemon juice

Directions:
1. Add all the above ingredients into your blender jar and pulse until thick and frothy.

Nutrition Info: (Per Serving): Calories- 234, Fat- 21 g, Protein- 3.3 g, Carbohydrates- 32 g

Bluberry Cucumber Cooler

Servings: 2
Cooking Time: 5 Minutes
Ingredients:
- 1 cup whole blueberries (fresh or frozen)
- 1 cup unsweetened almond milk
- ½ cup cucumber, chopped
- 2 large lettuce leaves
- 2 teaspoons hemp seeds
- 1 teaspoon raw organic honey (optional)
- 3-4 ice cubes

Directions:
1. Place all the ingredients into your blender and whirr it on high for 20 seconds or until the desired consistency has been reached. Pour into glasses and serve immediately.

Nutrition Info: (Per Serving): Calories- 202, Fat- 7.2 g, Protein- 6 g, Carbohydrates- 30 g

Saffron Oats Smoothie

Servings: 2-3
Cooking Time: 5 Minutes
Ingredients:
- 2 ripe banana, sliced (fresh or frozen)
- 1 cup fresh coconut water
- 1 teaspoon raw organic honey
- 2 tablespoons oats
- ½ teaspoon vanilla extract
- A pinch of saffron
- ½ teaspoon of almond or cashew flakes (optional)

Directions:
1. Place everything in the blender jar, secure the lid and pulse until smooth.

Nutrition Info: (Per Serving): Calories- 136, Fat- 1.2 g, Protein- 1.3 g, Carbohydrates- 33 g

Ultimate Super Food Smoothie

Servings: 3
Cooking Time: 5 Minutes
Ingredients:
- 1 cup unsweetened almond milk
- ¼ cup plain Greek yogurt
- ½ cup blueberries (fresh or frozen)
- ½ cup strawberries (fresh or frozen)
- 1 small ripe banana (fresh or frozen)
- A teaspoon coconut oil
- 1 ½ teaspoon bee pollen
- 1 teaspoon flax seeds
- 1 teaspoon Chia seed (soaked)
- 1 teaspoon fresh, pure Aloe Vera gel
- 1 teaspoon any other super food like maca, cacao, Hemp, Spirulina, wheatgrass, camu etc
- A few drops of liquid Stevia or agave nectar (optional)
- A pinch of cinnamon
- 4-5 ice cubes (optional)

Directions:
1. Whizz up all the ingredients in the high speed blender until smooth and serve immediately.

Nutrition Info: (Per Serving): Calories- 345, Fat- 17.6 g, Protein- 6.2 g, Carbohydrates- 45 g

Chocolate Shake Smoothie

Servings: 2
Cooking Time: 5 Minutes
Ingredients:
- 1 ½ cups unsweetened almond milk
- 6 teaspoons raw organic cacao powder
- 4 tablespoons Chia seeds, soaked
- 1 teaspoon vanilla extract
- 5 teaspoons raw, organic honey
- A small pinch of cinnamon powder
- 3-4 ice cubes

Directions:
1. Combine all the ingredients in your high speed blender and puree until it is thick and creamy.

Nutrition Info: (Per Serving): Calories- 428, Fat- 15 g, Protein- 10 g, Carbohydrates- 70 g

Mango-cado Blush

Servings: 2
Cooking Time: 5 Minutes
Ingredients:
- ½ cup freshly squeezed orange juice
- 1 cup mango, chopped
- 3 tablespoons ripe avocado flesh
- ¼ cup filtered water
- 1/3 cup loosely packed mint
- 2 teaspoons freshly squeezed lemon juice
- 2-3 ice cubes

Directions:
1. To your high speed blender, add all the items listed above and whip it on medium for 30 seconds or until well combined. Serve immediately.

Nutrition Info: (Per Serving): Calories- 145, Fat- 5.1, Protein- 2.2 g, Carbohydrates- 26 g

Kale And Pomegranate Smoothie

Servings: 3
Cooking Time: 5 Minutes
Ingredients:
- 2/3 cup freshly prepared pomegranate juice
- 1/3 cup unsweetened almond milk
- 1 cup fresh kale, stems removed and chopped
- ¼ cup blueberries (fresh or frozen)
- ¼ cup raspberries (fresh or frozen)
- 1 ripe banana, chopped
- A handful of mixed greens
- 1 tablespoon of hemp seeds
- 1 teaspoon agave nectar
- 1 cup filtered water
- 3-4 ice cubes

Directions:
1. Place all the above ingredients into the blender jar and process until the mixture is thick and creamy.

Nutrition Info: (Per Serving): Calories- 185, Fat- 0.5 g, Protein- 3.5 g, Carbohydrates- 40 g

All In 1 Smoothie

Servings: 2-3
Cooking Time: 5 Minutes
Ingredients:
- ½ cup freshly squeezed orange juice
- 1 cup carrots, peeled and chopped
- 1 cup fresh mixed greens of your choice
- 1 cup mixed berries (fresh or frozen)
- 1 small banana, copped (fresh or frozen)
- ½ cup plain low fat yogurt
- 2-3 drops of vanilla extract
- 1 teaspoon freshly squeezed lemon juice
- 3-4 ice cubes

Directions:
1. Pour all the ingredients into your blender and process until smooth.

Nutrition Info: (Per Serving): Calories- 160, Fat- 1.2 g, Protein- 5.3 g, Carbohydrates- 35 g

Pink Grapefruit Skin

Servings: 3
Cooking Time: 5 Minutes
Ingredients:
- 1 cups pineapple, chopped
- 1 small grapefruit, peeled and chopped
- 1 cups cucumber, chopped
- A handful of cilantro, washed and chopped
- ¾ cups freshly squeezed orange juice
- Freshly squeezed juice of ½ lime
- ½ teaspoon vanilla extract
- A pinch of cinnamon powder
- A pinch of sea salt
- ½ teaspoon raw organic honey
- 3-4 ice cubes

Directions:
1. Place all the above ingredients into the blender jar and process until the mixture is thick and creamy.

Nutrition Info: (Per Serving): Calories- 44, Fat- 0.5 g, Protein- 1 g, Carbohydrates- 9.1g

Pumpkin Spice Smoothie

Servings: 2
Cooking Time: 5 Minutes
Ingredients:
- 1 cup pumpkin, chopped

- ¾ cup plain yogurt
- 2 tablespoons avocado flesh
- 2 tablespoons flax seed powder
- ¼ pinch nutmeg powder
- A pinch of cinnamon powder
- A pinch of cayenne pepper
- ½ cup filtered water

Directions:
1. Pour all the items into the blender, secure the lid and blitz until the smoothie has reached a desired consistency and there are no lumps in the mixture. Pour into serving glasses and serve.

Nutrition Info: (Per Serving): Calories- 350, Fat- 15 g, Protein- 26 g, Carbohydrates- 39 g

Chocolaty Berry Blast

Servings: 2
Cooking Time: 2 Minutes
Ingredients:
- 2 cups unsweetened almond milk
- ½ cup Goji berries
- ½ cup whole almonds, soaked
- 6 teaspoons of raw cacao powder
- 1 tablespoon of raw organic honey
- 3-4 ice cubes

Directions:
1. To you blender, add all the above ingredient and pulse until smooth.

Nutrition Info: (Per Serving): Calories- 440, Fat- 23 g, Protein- 16 g, Carbohydrates- 43 g

Pink Potion

Servings: 3-4
Cooking Time: 5 Minutes
Ingredients:
- 2 cups raw beet, peeled and chopped
- 2 cups whole strawberries (fresh or frozen)
- 2 tablespoons almond butter
- 2 fresh kale leaves stems removed and chopped
- 1 banana, sliced (fresh or frozen)
- 1 teaspoon vanilla extract
- 1 tablespoon hemp seeds
- 1 cup filtered water

Directions:
1. Place all the ingredients into the blender and whiz up until the smoothie is nice and thick.

Nutrition Info: (Per Serving): Calories- 285, Fat- 11 g, Protein- 9.9 g, Carbohydrates- 40 g

Orange- Green Tonic

Servings: 1 Large
Cooking Time: 2 Minutes
Ingredients:
- ¾ cup mango, chopped
- ½ cup freshly squeezed orange juice
- ¾ cup fresh kale, stems removed and chopped
- 1-2 celery stalks, chopped
- 2 tablespoons fresh parsley
- 5-6 fresh mint
- 4-5 ice cubes

Directions:
1. Just add all the ingredients into the blender, secure the lid and whizz it up until nice and smooth.

Nutrition Info: (Per Serving): Calories- 160, Fat- 0.7 g, Protein- 4.3 g, Carbohydrates- 38.5 g

Grape And Strawberry Smoothie

Servings: 2
Cooking Time: 5 Minutes
Ingredients:
- ½ cup whole strawberries (fresh or frozen)
- ½ cup red grapes, seedless
- 1 cup baby spinach, washed
- 1 cup mixed greens
- 2 tablespoons avocado flesh
- 2 teaspoons almond butter
- 1 teaspoon flax seed powder
- ¼ cup freshly squeezed lemon juice
- ¾ cup filtered water
- 2-3 ice cubes

Directions:
1. Whizz all the ingredients in the blender until smooth and serve.

Nutrition Info: (Per Serving): Calories- 310, Fat- 2 g, Protein- 8 g, Carbohydrates- 26 g

Crunchy Kale – Chia Smoothie

Servings: 3-4
Cooking Time: 5 Minutes
Ingredients:
- 1 cup fresh kale, stems removed and chopped
- A large handful of strawberries (fresh or frozen)
- A large handful of raspberries (fresh or frozen)
- ¼ cup red bell pepper, deseeded and chopped
- 1 ½ cups unsweetened almond milk
- 1 cup fresh coconut water
- 1 ½ teaspoon Chia seeds
- 6-7 whole almonds, soaked

Directions:
1. Add all the above ingredients into your blender jar and pulse until thick and frothy.

Nutrition Info: (Per Serving): Calories- 234, Fat- 21.5 g, Protein- 3 g, Carbohydrates- 21 g

Nutty Raspberry Avocado Blend

Servings: 2
Cooking Time: 5 Minutes
Ingredients:
- 1 cup whole raspberries (fresh or frozen)
- 3/4 cup avocado, peeled, pitted and chopped
- 3/4 cup cashews, soaked
- 1 tablespoon organic coconut oil
- 1 ½ - 2 cups filtered water
- A pinch of Himalayan salt

Directions:
1. Dump all the ingredients into the blender and whip it up until the smoothie is thick and creamy.

Nutrition Info: (Per Serving): Calories- 698, Fat- 54 g, Protein- 9.1 g, Carbohydrates- 53 g

Berry Beautiful Glowing Skin Smoothie

Servings: 2
Cooking Time: 5 Minutes
Ingredients:
- 1 cup blueberries (fresh or frozen)
- ½ cup raspberries (fresh or frozen)
- ½ cup strawberries (fresh or frozen)
- A handful of fresh kale, stems removed and chopped
- ¾ cup of plain Greek yogurt
- 2 teaspoon of raw organic honey
- 2 teaspoons freshly squeezed lemon juice
- 3 teaspoons flaxseed powder
- 4-5 ice cubes

Directions:
1. Pour all the ingredients into your blender and process until smooth.

Nutrition Info: (Per Serving): Calories- 161, Fat- 1.3 g, Protein- 8.9 g, Carbohydrates- 32 g

Cantaloupe Yogurt Smoothie

Servings: 1 Large
Cooking Time: 2 Minutes
Ingredients:
- 1 cup cantaloupe, chopped
- 1/3 cup plain yogurt
- ¼ teaspoon freshly grated ginger
- A pinch of nutmeg powder
- 1 tablespoon raw organic honey
- 1 teaspoon freshly squeezed lemon juice
- 3-4 mint leaves
- ½ cup filtered water
- 6-7 ice cubes

Directions:
1. Place everything into a blender and blitz until smooth. Pour into a glass and enjoy!

Nutrition Info: (Per Serving): Calories- 90, Fat- 0.9 g, Protein- 3.1 g, Carbohydrates- 20 g

Aloe Berry Smoothie

Servings: 2
Cooking Time: 2 Minutes
Ingredients:
- ½ cup blueberries (fresh or frozen)
- 1/3 cup fresh and pure aloe gel or aloe Vera juice
- 2 tablespoons avocado flesh
- A handful of dandelion greens, chopped
- 1 kiwi, peeled and chopped
- 1 teaspoon coconut oil
- 1 teaspoon cacao powder
- A pinch of Celtic salt
- 1 ½ teaspoons of raw organic honey
- 1 cup filtered water

Directions:
1. Combine all the ingredients in a blender, secure the lid firmly and blitz until smooth.

Nutrition Info: (Per Serving): Calories- 305, Fat- 15 g, Protein- 2.1 g, Carbohydrates- 45 g

ENERGY BOOSTING SMOOTHIES

Pumpkin Seed And Yogurt Smoothie

Servings: 2
Cooking Time: 5 Minutes
Ingredients:
- 1 cup plain Greek yogurt
- 1 cup freshly squeezed grapefruit juice
- 1 avocado, peeled, pitted and chopped
- 2 cups fresh kale, stems removed
- 3 teaspoons almond butter
- 3 teaspoons pumpkin seeds
- ½ cup filtered water

Directions:
1. Add all the ingredients into the blender jar and whirr it up until nice and smooth.

Nutrition Info: (Per Serving): Calories- 432, Fat- 32 g, Protein- 17g, Carbohydrates- 42 g

Green Skinny Energizer

Servings: 2
Cooking Time: 5 Minutes
Ingredients:
- ½ ripe mango, pitted and sliced
- 1 cup kale, chopped
- 3 cups baby spinach
- 1 cup coconut water

Directions:
1. Add all the ingredients except vegetables/fruits first
2. Blend until smooth
3. Add the vegetable/fruits
4. Blend until smooth
5. Add a few ice cubes and serve the smoothie
6. Enjoy!

Nutrition Info: Calories: 300; Fat: 13g; Carbohydrates: 37g; Protein: 10g

Avocado Wonder Smoothie

Servings: 2 Large
Cooking Time: 5 Minutes
Ingredients:
- 2 cups unsweetened almond milk
- 1 large ripe avocado, peeled, pitted and chopped
- A small handful of spinach, chopped
- 3 teaspoons of raw organic honey
- 1 teaspoon freshly squeezed lemon juice
- 4-5 ice cubes

Directions:
1. Place all the smoothie ingredients into the blender and puree whirr it up until everything is well combined.

Nutrition Info: (Per Serving): Calories-301, Fat- 20 g, Protein- 10 g, Carbohydrates- 23.9 g

Orange Antioxidant Refresher

Servings: 2
Cooking Time: 5 Minutes
Ingredients:
- 4 ounces pineapple
- 1 orange, peeled
- 1 teaspoon pomegranate powder
- 1 mini orange, peeled
- ½ teaspoon turmeric
- ½ teaspoon ginger
- 1 cup ice
- 1 cup of water

Directions:
1. Add all the listed ingredients to a blender
2. Blend until you have a smooth and creamy texture
3. Serve chilled and enjoy!

Nutrition Info: Calories: 101; Fat: 1g; Carbohydrates: 25g; Protein: 2g

Persimmon Pineapple Protein Smoothie

Servings: 2
Cooking Time: 5 Minutes
Ingredients:
- 1 persimmon, topped and chopped
- 1 tablespoon cinnamon
- 1 squash
- 1 tablespoon flaxseed
- 4 ounces pineapple
- 1 tablespoon pea protein
- 1 cup of water

Directions:
1. Add all the listed ingredients to a blender
2. Blend until you have a smooth and creamy texture
3. Serve chilled and enjoy!

Nutrition Info: Calories: 159; Fat: 2g; Carbohydrates: 33g; Protein: 7g

Almond-banana Booster

Servings: 2
Cooking Time: 5 Minutes
Ingredients:
- 2 large banana, chopped (fresh or frozen)
- 1 cup unsweetened almond milk
- A handful of almonds

- ¼ cup plain Greek yogurt
- 2 tablespoons Chia seeds, soaked
- 1 teaspoon hemp seed powder
- 2 teaspoons freshly squeezed lemon juice
- 1 teaspoon raw organic honey
- A handful of ice cubes

Directions:
1. Pour everything into the blender and process for 30 seconds until nice and thick.

Nutrition Info: (Per Serving): Calories- 244, Fat- 6.2 g, Protein- 7 g, Carbohydrates- 32 g

Mango Honey Smoothie

Servings: 2
Cooking Time: 10 Minutes
Ingredients:
- 2 mangoes, peeled, pit removed and chopped
- 4 teaspoons honey
- 3 cups almond milk
- 16 ice cubes

Directions:
1. Add all the listed ingredients to a blender
2. Blend until you have a smooth and creamy texture
3. Serve chilled and enjoy!

Nutrition Info: Calories: 223; Fat: 3.4g; Carbohydrates: 49.2g; Protein: 2.9g

Powerful Green Frenzy

Servings: 2
Cooking Time: 5 Minutes
Ingredients:
- 1 cup ice
- 2 tablespoons almond butter
- 1 teaspoon spirulina
- 3 teaspoons fresh ginger
- 1½ frozen bananas, sliced
- 2 cups baby spinach, chopped
- 1 cup kale
- 1½ cups unsweetened almond milk

Directions:
1. Add all the ingredients except vegetables/fruits first
2. Blend until smooth
3. Add the vegetable/fruits
4. Blend until smooth
5. Add a few ice cubes and serve the smoothie
6. Enjoy!

Nutrition Info: Calories: 350; Fat: 4g; Carbohydrates: 54g; Protein: 30g

Ginger- Pomegranate Smoothie

Servings: 2
Cooking Time: 2 Minutes
Ingredients:
- 1 cup freshly prepared homemade pomegranate juice
- 4 ounces of plain Greek yogurt
- 1 large banana, chopped (fresh or frozen)
- ¼ teaspoon freshly grated ginger
- 1 teaspoon freshly squeezed lemon juice
- 3-4 ice cubes

Directions:
1. Pour all the ingredients into the blender and puree until smooth and frothy.

Nutrition Info: (Per Serving): Calories- 192, Fat- 2.1 g, Protein- 7.8 g, Carbohydrates- 40 g

Berry Flax Smoothie

Servings: 4
Cooking Time: 10 Minutes
Ingredients:
- 3 cups dairy-free milk
- 2 cups spinach
- 2 tablespoons flaxseeds, ground
- 1 cup berries, fresh or frozen
- 2 teaspoons ginger root, peeled

Directions:
1. Add all the listed ingredients to a blender
2. Blend until you have a smooth and creamy texture
3. Serve chilled and enjoy!

Nutrition Info: Calories: 212; Fat: 11.9g; Carbohydrates: 31.7g; Protein: 7.3g

Coconut-banana Smoothie

Servings: 2-3
Cooking Time: 5 Minutes
Ingredients:
- 1 cup fresh coconut milk
- 1 teaspoon almond butter
- 2 cups spinach, washed and chopped
- large banana, chopped (fresh or frozen)
- ½ teaspoon raw, organic honey
- 1 teaspoon flax seed powder
- 3-4 ice cubes

Directions:
1. Combine all the ingredients in the high speed blender jar and blend until done.

Nutrition Info: (Per Serving): Calories- 135, Fat- 8.2 g, Protein- 4 g, Carbohydrates- 21 g

Dandelion And Carrot Booster

Servings: 2
Cooking Time: 5 Minutes
Ingredients:
- ½ fuji apple
- 1 tablespoon fresh ginger
- ½ pound organic carrots, scrubbed
- ¾ cup dandelion greens
- 2 cups baby spinach

Directions:
1. Add all the ingredients except vegetables/fruits first
2. Blend until smooth
3. Add the vegetable/fruits
4. Blend until smooth
5. Add a few ice cubes and serve the smoothie
6. Enjoy!

Nutrition Info: Calories: 160; Fat: 5g; Carbohydrates: 30g; Protein: 5g

Verry- Berry Breakfast

Servings: 2
Cooking Time: 2 Minutes
Ingredients:
- ¾ cup unsweetened almond milk
- ½ large banana, chopped
- ¾ cup plain Greek yogurt
- 1 cup mixed berries (fresh or frozen)
- ½ teaspoon raw organic honey (optional)
- 3-5 ice cubes

Directions:
1. Place all the above ingredients into your high speed blender and process for 45 seconds on medium high speed till the smoothie is thick and creamy.

Nutrition Info: (Per Serving): Calories- 255, Fat- 1.2 g, Protein- 26 g, Carbohydrates- 42 g

Apple- Date Smoothie

Servings: 3
Cooking Time: 5 Minutes
Ingredients:
- 2 large apples, peeled, cored and chopped
- 1 large ripe banana, chopped
- 3 tablespoons almond butter or cashew butter
- 4-5 collard greens, stems removed and chopped
- 2-3 medjool dates, pitted
- 3 teaspoons hemp powder
- 1 ½ cups filtered water

Directions:
1. Place all the ingredients into your high speed blender jar and pulse it for 30 seconds until everything is well combined.

Nutrition Info: (Per Serving): Calories- 481, Fat- 20 g, Protein- 12.2 g, Carbohydrates- 73.5 g

Awesome Pineapple And Carrot Blend

Servings: 2
Cooking Time: 5 Minutes
Ingredients:
- 1/8 teaspoon cinnamon
- 1 cup fresh pineapple
- 3 organic carrots, scrubbed and sliced
- 5 cups baby spinach
- 1 large cucumber, diced

Directions:
1. Add all the ingredients except vegetables/fruits first
2. Blend until smooth
3. Add the vegetable/fruits
4. Blend until smooth
5. Add a few ice cubes and serve the smoothie
6. Enjoy!

Nutrition Info: Calories: 82; Fat: 0g; Carbohydrates: 21g; Protein: 1g

Goji Berry- Pineapple Wonder

Servings: 2-3
Cooking Time: 2 Minutes
Ingredients:
- ½ cup pineapple, chipped
- ½ cup mango, chopped
- 1 cup fresh coconut water
- ¼ cup loosely packed arugula leaves
- ¼ cup loosely packed parsley
- 1/3 cup goji berries, soaked
- 3 teaspoons organic coconut oil
- 1 teaspoon bee pollen (optional)
- 1-2 celery leaves or stalks
- 3 teaspoons fresh coconut flakes

Directions:
1. To your blender, place all the above listed items and run it on high for 30 seconds or until smooth.

Nutrition Info: (Per Serving): Calories- 462, Fat- 28 g, Protein- 5.4 g, Carbohydrates- 55 g

Oats And Blueberry Smoothie

Servings: X
Cooking Time: 2 Minutes
Ingredients:

- 2/3 cup blueberries (frozen or fresh)
- ½ cup unsweetened almond milk
- 1/3 cup plain yogurt
- 1 medium banana. Chopped
- 2-3 drops of vanilla extract
- 2 teaspoon rolled oats
- A pinch of cinnamon powder
- 4-5 ice cubes

Directions:
1. Combine all the ingredients in your blender and puree for 45 seconds. Pour into servings glasses and enjoy.

Nutrition Info: (Per Serving): Calories- 274, Fat- 5 g, Protein- 10 g, Carbohydrates- 47 g

Cinnamon Mango Smoothie

Servings: 2
Cooking Time: 10 Minutes
Ingredients:
- 2 mangoes, peeled, pit removed and chopped
- ½ teaspoon cinnamon, grounded
- 2 teaspoons lime juice
- 2 cups plain yogurt, low-fat
- 1 tablespoon honey

Directions:
1. Add all the listed ingredients to a blender
2. Blend until you have a smooth and creamy texture
3. Serve chilled and enjoy!

Nutrition Info: Calories: 210; Fat: 2.2g; Carbohydrates: 40.2g; Protein: 8.5g

Coco- Cranberry Smoothie

Servings: 3
Cooking Time: 5 Minutes
Ingredients:
- 1 cup fresh coconut water
- ½ green avocado, peeled and chopped
- ¼ cup mango, chopped
- ½ cup fresh spinach, chopped
- ½ cup kale, stems removed and chopped
- ¼ cup papaya, chopped
- 1/3 cup plain yogurt
- ¼ cup cranberries(fresh , frozen or dried)
- ¼ cup Goji berries
- 1 teaspoon wheatgrass powder
- 1 tablespoon maca root powder
- 1 teaspoon pure coconut oil
- 1 teaspoon raw, organic honey

Directions:
1. Add all the ingredients one by one into your blender jar, secure the lid and run it on high for 30 seconds or until done.

Nutrition Info: (Per Serving): Calories- 531, Fat- 32 g, Protein- 15 g, Carbohydrates- 65 g

Banana Apple Blast

Servings: 2
Cooking Time: 5 Minutes
Ingredients:
- 1 cup ice
- 1 teaspoon bee pollen
- 1 teaspoon spirulina
- 1 cup fresh pineapple, sliced
- 1 frozen banana, sliced
- 2 cups baby spinach
- 1½ cups unsweetened coconut milk drink

Directions:
1. Add all the ingredients except vegetables/fruits first
2. Blend until smooth
3. Add the vegetable/fruits
4. Blend until smooth
5. Add a few ice cubes and serve the smoothie
6. Enjoy!

Nutrition Info: Calories: 209; Fat: 2g; Carbohydrates: 51g; Protein: 2g

Generous Mango Surprise

Servings: 2
Cooking Time: 5 Minutes
Ingredients:
- 1 tablespoon spirulina
- 3 cups frozen mango, sliced
- 1½ cups kale
- 2½ cups unsweetened almond milk

Directions:
1. Add all the ingredients except vegetables/fruits first
2. Blend until smooth
3. Add the vegetable/fruits
4. Blend until smooth
5. Add a few ice cubes and serve the smoothie
6. Enjoy!

Nutrition Info: Calories: 72; Fat: 0g; Carbohydrates: 17g; Protein: 1g

Pumpkin Power Smoothie

Servings: 2
Cooking Time: 10 Minutes
Ingredients:

- 2 cups pumpkin puree
- 2 pumpkin pie spice, dashes
- 1 banana, frozen
- 2 dashes pie spice, dashes
- 2 handfuls ice cubes

Directions:
1. Add all the listed ingredients to a blender
2. Blend until you have a smooth and creamy texture
3. Serve chilled and enjoy!

Nutrition Info: Calories: 177; Fat: 3.9g; Carbohydrates: 35.3g; Protein: 4.4g

Coco-nana Smoothie

Servings: 1 Large
Cooking Time: 2 Minutes
Ingredients:
- ¾ cup fresh coconut water
- A handful of whole strawberries (fresh or frozen)
- 1 ripe banana (fresh or frozen)
- A handful of spinach leaves
- 1 teaspoon of flax seed powder
- 2-3 ice cubes (optional)

Directions:
1. Pour all the ingredients in the blender and pulse until there are no lumps. Pour into glasses and enjoy.

Nutrition Info: (Per Serving): Calories- 145, Fat- 2.2 g, Protein- 3.1 g, Carbohydrates- 32 g

Peppermint Stick Smoothie

Servings: 2
Cooking Time: 5 Minutes
Ingredients:
- 1 banana, peeled
- 1 tablespoon coconut milk
- 4 spring mint
- 1 and ½ tablespoons cacao powder
- 1 apple, chopped
- 1 cup ice
- 1 cup of water

Directions:
1. Add all the listed ingredients to a blender
2. Blend until you have a smooth and creamy texture
3. Serve chilled and enjoy!

Nutrition Info: Calories: 150; Fat: 5g; Carbohydrates: 29g; Protein: 2g

Powerful Purple Smoothie

Servings: 2
Cooking Time: 5 Minutes
Ingredients:
- 1 tablespoon green superfood as you like
- 1 tablespoon spirulina
- 1 frozen banana, sliced
- 2 acai frozen berry packs
- 2 cups baby spinach
- 1¼ cups of coconut water

Directions:
1. Add all the ingredients except vegetables/fruits first
2. Blend until smooth
3. Add the vegetable/fruits
4. Blend until smooth
5. Add a few ice cubes and serve the smoothie
6. Enjoy!

Nutrition Info: Calories: 70; Fat: 2g; Carbohydrates: 14g; Protein: 3g

Mct Strawberry Smoothie

Servings: 2
Cooking Time: 10 Minutes
Ingredients:
- 1 and ¼ cups of coconut milk
- 4 tablespoons strawberry
- ½ cup heavy whipping cream
- 14 large ice cubes
- ½ teaspoon xanthan gum
- 2 tablespoons MCT oil

Directions:
1. Add all the listed ingredients to a blender
2. Blend until you have a smooth and creamy texture
3. Serve chilled and enjoy!

Nutrition Info: Calories: 373; Fat: 45.1g; Carbohydrates: 5.8g; Protein: 2.1g

Coconut- Flaxseed Smoothie

Servings: 1
Cooking Time: 2 Minutes
Ingredients:
- 1 cup fresh coconut water
- 1 small bananas, chopped
- 4 spinach leaves, washed and chopped
- ½ cup whole strawberries (fresh or frozen)
- 1 tablespoon flaxseed powder
- 3-4 ice cubes

Directions:
1. Load all the ingredients into the blender and whiz until smooth.

Nutrition Info: (Per Serving): Calories- 300, Fat- 4.2 g, Protein- 6.2 g, Carbohydrates- 67 g

Mango Beet Energy Booster

Servings: 2
Cooking Time: 5 Minutes
Ingredients:
- ½ cup unsweetened almond milk
- 1 cup red beet, peeled and chopped
- 1 ripe banana, chopped (fresh or frozen)
- 1 small mango, peeled and chopped
- 2 cups baby spinach, chopped
- ½ teaspoon freshly grated giber
- A handful of ice cubes

Directions:
1. Load your blender with all the ingredients mentioned above and run it on medium high for 45 seconds until there are no lumps. Pour into beautiful glasses and serve.

Nutrition Info: (Per Serving): Calories- 165, Fat- 1.1 g, Protein- 4 g, Carbohydrates- 40 g

Mango Energizer

Servings: 2
Cooking Time: 5 Minutes
Ingredients:
- 4 tablespoons protein powder
- 2 teaspoons spirulina
- 1 teaspoon bee pollen
- 1 frozen banana, sliced
- 1 cup frozen mango, sliced
- 2 cups baby spinach
- 1¼ cups unsweetened almond milk

Directions:
1. Add all the ingredients except vegetables/fruits first
2. Blend until smooth
3. Add the vegetable/fruits
4. Blend until smooth
5. Add a few ice cubes and serve the smoothie
6. Enjoy!

Nutrition Info: Calories: 136; Fat: 2g; Carbohydrates: 29g; Protein: 5g

Berry- Mint Cooler

Servings: 2
Cooking Time: 2 Minutes
Ingredients:
- 2 cups unsweetened almond milk
- A large handful of frozen blueberries
- 1 ½ teaspoons of raw, organic honey
- 1 ½ teaspoon flax seed powder
- 3-4 fresh mint leaves
- 4-5 ice cubes

Directions:
1. To your high speed blender, add all the ingredients and process for 30 seconds or until done.

Nutrition Info: (Per Serving): Calories- 201, Fat-7.2 g, Protein-11 g, Carbohydrates- 21 g

DIABETES SMOOTHIES

Green Tea And Carrot Smoothie

Servings: 2
Cooking Time: 25 Minutes
Ingredients:
- ½ cup carrots, peeled and sliced
- 2 green tea bags
- 1 cup mango, chopped (fresh or frozen)
- ½ teaspoon freshly grated ginger
- 1 teaspoon Chia sees, soaked
- ½ teaspoon raw organic honey
- 1 ½ cup filtered water
- 1 teaspoon freshly squeezed lemon juice

Directions:
1. Boil the water in a sauce pan and cook the carrot until they are tender.
2. Add the ginger into the saucepan, just a few minutes before turning off the heat, after you put off the flame, place the tea bags in the same sauce pan and let it steep for a few minutes.
3. One the tea has infused into the water, remove the tea bags and allow the green tea carrot mixture to cool to room temperature.
4. Transfer the contents from the sauce pan into the blender along with all the remaining ingredients and blend until thick and smooth.

Nutrition Info: (Per Serving): Calories- 70, Fat- 0 g, Protein- 1.1 g, Carbohydrates- 12 g

Hemp And Kale Smoothie

Servings: 2
Cooking Time: 5 Minutes
Ingredients:
- 1 large banana, chopped (fresh or frozen)
- A large handful of baby spinach, washed and chopped
- A large handful of kale, stems removed and chopped
- 1 tablespoon of hemp seeds
- 2-3 drops of liquid Stevia (optional)
- 2 teaspoons of freshly squeezed lemon juice
- 1 ½ cups of filtered water

Directions:
1. Place all the ingredients in the blender jar, secure the lid and pulse it for 20 seconds until everything is well combined.

Nutrition Info: (Per Serving): Calories- 340, Fat- 16 g, Protein- 15 g, Carbohydrates- 44 g

Cashew Apple Glass

Servings: 2
Cooking Time: 5 Minutes
Ingredients:
- 1 cup ice
- 1 teaspoon apple pie spice
- 1 tablespoon cashew butter
- 1 medium apple, peeled and chopped
- ½ cup frozen peaches
- 1 serving whey protein powder
- ¾ cup plain soymilk

Directions:
1. Add all the ingredients except vegetables/fruits first
2. Blend until smooth
3. Add the vegetable/fruits
4. Blend until smooth
5. Add a few ice cubes and serve the smoothie
6. Enjoy!

Nutrition Info: Calories: 500; Fat: 17g; Carbohydrates: 63g; Protein: 9g

Plum- Bokchoy Smoothie

Servings: 2
Cooking Time: 5 Minutes
Ingredients:
- 1 cup kale, stems removed and chopped
- 1 banana, chopped (fresh or frozen)
- 1 medium head bok choy
- 1 large red plum, pitted and chopped
- 2 tablespoons avocado flesh
- 2 teaspoons freshly squeezed lime juice
- ½ cup filtered water
- 2-3 ice cubes

Directions:
1. Load the high speed bender with all the ingredients and pulse until smooth.

Nutrition Info: (Per Serving): Calories- 260, Fat-10 g, Protein- 8 g, Carbohydrates- 45 g

Healthy Potato Pie Glass

Servings: 2
Cooking Time: 5 Minutes
Ingredients:
- 1 cup ice
- ¼ teaspoon cinnamon
- ¼ cup rolled oats
- ½ frozen banana
- 1 small orange, peeled
- ½ cup sweet potato, cooked and peeled
- 6 ounces Greek yogurt
- ½ cup unsweetened almond milk

Directions:
1. Add all the ingredients except vegetables/fruits first
2. Blend until smooth
3. Add the vegetable/fruits
4. Blend until smooth
5. Add a few ice cubes and serve the smoothie
6. Enjoy!

Nutrition Info: Calories: 400; Fat: 20g; Carbohydrates: 41g; Protein: 20g

Spicy Pear And Green Tea

Servings: 2
Cooking Time: 5 Minutes
Ingredients:
- 1 cup brewed and chilled green tea
- ½ cup silken tofu
- 1 small pear, skin on, cut into small pieces
- ½ frozen bananas, sliced into rounds
- 2 tablespoons ground flaxseed
- 1/8 teaspoon cayenne
- 2 tablespoons lemon juice
- ½ cup ice

Directions:
1. Add all the ingredients except vegetables/fruits first
2. Blend until smooth
3. Add the vegetable/fruits
4. Blend until smooth
5. Add a few ice cubes and serve the smoothie
6. Enjoy!

Nutrition Info: Calories: 422; Fat: 13g; Carbohydrates: 51g; Protein: 31g

Avocado Turmeric Smoothie

Servings: 1
Cooking Time: 10 Minutes
Ingredients:
- 1 avocado
- 2 teaspoons lemon juice
- 1 teaspoon turmeric
- 2 teaspoons ginger, fresh grated
- 1 and ¼ cups of coconut milk
- 2 cups ice, crushed
- Stevia, to taste

Directions:
1. Add all the listed ingredients to a blender
2. Blend until you have a smooth and creamy texture
3. Serve chilled and enjoy!

Nutrition Info: Calories: 320; Fat: 27.4g; Carbohydrates: 11g; Protein: 4.3g

Tropical Kiwi Pineapple

Servings: 2
Cooking Time: 5 Minutes
Ingredients:
- 1 cup ice
- 1 tablespoon ground flaxseed
- 1 tablespoon psyllium husk
- 6 almonds
- 2 tablespoons unsweetened coconut
- 1 medium kiwi, skin intact

Directions:
1. Add all the ingredients except vegetables/fruits first
2. Blend until smooth
3. Add the vegetable/fruits
4. Blend until smooth
5. Add a few ice cubes and serve the smoothie
6. Enjoy!

Nutrition Info: Calories: 300; Fat: 15g; Carbohydrates: 40g; Protein: 1g

Coconut Pear Crunch Smoothie

Servings: 2
Cooking Time: 2 Minutes
Ingredients:
- 1 cup fresh coconut milk
- 1 medium pear, cored and chopped
- 1 large apple, Cored and chopped
- 1 teaspoon Chia seeds
- 10 -12 unsalted whole almonds

Directions:
1. Load the blender with all the ingredients listed above and blend until smooth.

Nutrition Info: (Per Serving): Calories- 195, Fat- 5 g, Protein- 4.2 g, Carbohydrates- 45 g

Cucumber-kale Chiller

Servings: 2
Cooking Time: 5 Minutes
Ingredients:
- 1 cup fresh coconut milk
- ½ cup cucumber, chopped
- ½ cup pineapple, chopped
- 2 kiwi frits, peeled and chopped
- 2/3 cup fresh kale, stems removed and chopped
- 2 tablespoon freshly squeezed lime juice
- 1 teaspoon freshly squeezed lemon juice
- 3-4 ice cubes

Directions:

1. Place all the above listed items in the blender jar, secure the lid and whizz until smooth.
Nutrition Info: (Per Serving): Calories- 106, Fat- 6.5 g, Protein-5 g, Carbohydrates- 53 g

Greens And Herbs For All

Servings: 2
Cooking Time: 5 Minutes
Ingredients:
- 1 cup ice
- 1 tablespoon ground flaxseed
- 1/3 cup fresh cilantro, chopped
- ½ lemon, juiced
- 1 pear, cored and chopped
- ½ frozen banana, sliced into rounds
- 2 cups baby spinach, chopped
- 2 stalks celery, chopped
- 1 cup romaine lettuce, chopped
- ½ cup non-fat Greek yogurt
- 1 cup water

Directions:
1. Add all the ingredients except vegetables/fruits first
2. Blend until smooth
3. Add the vegetable/fruits
4. Blend until smooth
5. Add a few ice cubes and serve the smoothie
6. Enjoy!

Nutrition Info: Calories: 184; Fat: 1g; Carbohydrates: 45g; Protein: 6g

Diabetic Berry Blast

Servings: 1
Cooking Time: 10 Minutes
Ingredients:
- 2 tablespoons flax meal
- 3 kale leaves
- 2 cups unsweetened mango chunks
- 1 cup frozen raspberries
- 1 cup frozen blackberries
- 1 cup frozen blueberries

Directions:
1. Add all the listed ingredients to a blender
2. Blend until you have a smooth and creamy texture
3. Serve chilled and enjoy!

Nutrition Info: Calories: 153; Fat: 11g; Carbohydrates: 8g; Protein: 7g

Oat, Celery Green Smoothie

Servings: 2
Cooking Time: 5 Minutes
Ingredients:
- ¾ cup unsweetened almond milk
- ¼ cup tightly packed spinach, washed and chopped
- ¼ cup cucumber, chopped
- ½ cup whole strawberries (fresh or frozen)
- ¼ cup whole strawberries (fresh or frozen)
- 1 celery stalk, chopped
- 4 teaspoons rolled oats
- 1 ½ teaspoon cacao powder
- 1 ½ teaspoon flax seed powder
- ½ teaspoon cinnamon powder
- 4-5 ice cubes

Directions:
1. Load your blender jar with the above listed items and process until smooth.

Nutrition Info: (Per Serving): Calories- 340, Fat- 12.3 g, Protein- 13.1 g, Carbohydrates- 47 g

Lime "n" Lemony Cucumber Cooler

Servings: 3
Cooking Time: 5 Minutes
Ingredients:
- 2 cups plain fat free yogurt
- 2 cups green cucumber, chopped
- 1 green pear, cored and chopped
- Freshly squeezed juice of 1 lime
- 1 tablespoon freshly squeezed lemon juice
- 2-3 ice cubes

Directions:
1. Place all the ingredients into the high speed blender and blitz until thick and creamy. Serve immediately!

Nutrition Info: (Per Serving): Calories- 175, Fat- 4.2 g, Protein- 11 g, Carbohydrates- 63 g

Berry-licious Meta Booster

Servings: 2
Cooking Time: 5 Minutes
Ingredients:
- ¼ cup garbanzo bean
- 1 teaspoon flax oil
- ½ cup frozen blueberries
- ½ cup frozen broccoli florets
- 6 ounces Greek yogurt
- ¾ cup brewed and chilled green tea

Directions:
1. Add all the ingredients except vegetables/fruits first
2. Blend until smooth
3. Add the vegetable/fruits
4. Blend until smooth
5. Add a few ice cubes and serve the smoothie
6. Enjoy!

Nutrition Info: Calories: 200; Fat: 3g; Carbohydrates: 41g; Protein: 5g

Peanut Butter And Raspberry Delight

Servings: 2
Cooking Time: 5 Minutes
Ingredients:
- 1 tablespoon psyllium husk
- 1 tablespoon unsweetened peanut butter
- 2 tablespoons powdered peanut butter
- ¾ cup frozen cherries
- ½ cup silken tofu
- ¾ cup non-fat milk such as almond milk

Directions:
1. Add all the ingredients except vegetables/fruits first
2. Blend until smooth
3. Add the vegetable/fruits
4. Blend until smooth
5. Add a few ice cubes and serve the smoothie
6. Enjoy!

Nutrition Info: Calories: 170; Fat: 8g; Carbohydrates: 24g; Protein: 6g

Berry Truffle Smoothie

Servings: 2
Cooking Time: 10 Minutes
Ingredients:
- 1 medium Haas avocado
- 1 and ¼ teaspoons pure vanilla extract
- ½ cup whipping cream
- 3 tablespoons cocoa powder, unsweetened
- 4 tablespoons pecans
- 1 and ¼ cups mixed berries, frozen
- 2 pinches salt
- ¾ cups of ice cubes
- Erythritol, to taste
- 1 cup of water

Directions:
1. Add all the listed ingredients to a blender
2. Blend until you have a smooth and creamy texture
3. Serve chilled and enjoy!

Nutrition Info: Calories: 375; Fat: 32.5g; Carbohydrates: 11.3g; Protein: 5.8g

Keto Mocha Smoothie

Servings: 4
Cooking Time: 10 Minutes
Ingredients:
- 6 tablespoons cocoa powder, unsweetened
- 1 cup of coconut milk
- 3 cups almond milk, unsweetened
- 2 avocados, cut in half
- 2 teaspoons vanilla extract
- 6 tablespoons erythritol, granulated
- 4 teaspoons instant coffee crystals

Directions:

1. Add all the listed ingredients to a blender
2. Blend until you have a smooth and creamy texture
3. Serve chilled and enjoy!

Nutrition Info: Calories: 273; Fat: 24.3g; Carbohydrates: 8.2g; Protein: 4.5g

Triple Berry Delight

Servings: 2 Servings
Cooking Time: 2 Minutes
Ingredients:
- ½ cup freshly prepared pomegranate juice
- ½ cup blackberries (fresh or frozen)
- ½ cup raspberries (fresh or frozen)
- 1 cup whole strawberries (fresh or frozen)
- ½ cup baby spinach, washed and chopped
- 1 teaspoon freshly squeezed lemon juice
- 3-4 ice cubes

Directions:
1. Pour the ingredients into your high speed blender and run it on high for 20 seconds or until everything is well combined. Serve immediately.

Nutrition Info: (Per Serving): Calories- 120, Fat- 1 g, Protein- 5.2 g, Carbohydrates- 27 g

Avocado And Edamame Drink

Servings: 2
Cooking Time: 5 Minutes
Ingredients:
- ¾ cup almond milk
- ½ cup edamame shelled
- ¼ cup avocado, diced
- ½ cup of frozen mango, diced
- 1 tablespoon coconut flour
- 1 cup ice

Directions:
1. Add all the ingredients except vegetables/fruits first
2. Blend until smooth
3. Add the vegetable/fruits
4. Blend until smooth
5. Add a few ice cubes and serve the smoothie
6. Enjoy!

Nutrition Info: Calories: 245; Fat: 15g; Carbohydrates: 28g; Protein: 4g

Cashew- Goji Berry Smoothie

Servings: 2 -3
Cooking Time: 5 Minutes
Ingredients:
- ½ cup whole cashew nuts
- ½ cup pineapple, peeled and chopped
- ½ cup whole strawberries (fresh or frozen)

- 1 cup Swiss chard leaves (stems removed and chopped)
- 1 cup kale, washed and chopped
- 1/3 cup Goji berries
- ½ cup plain Greek yogurt
- ½ cup filtered water

Directions:
1. Combine all the ingredients in the blender and whip it up until nice and smooth.

Nutrition Info: (Per Serving): Calories- 385, Fat- 15 g, Protein- 16 g, Carbohydrates- 56 g

Coconut -mint Smoothie

Servings: 2
Cooking Time: 5 Minutes
Ingredients:
- 1 cup mango, chopped
- 1 cup fresh kale, stems removed and chopped
- A handful of lettuce
- 1-2 celery stalks
- ½ cup fresh mint, washed and chopped
- ½ cup Italian flat leafed parsley, washed
- 2 teaspoon coconut oil
- ¾ cup coconut water

Directions:
1. Place everything into the blender, secure the lid and process until smooth.

Nutrition Info: (Per Serving): Calories-220, Fat- 15 g, 4.1 g, Protein- Carbohydrates- 25 g

Pineapple Broccoli Smoothie

Servings: 2
Cooking Time: 10 Minutes
Ingredients:
- 1 cup strawberries
- 2 cups almond milk
- 2 cups broccoli florets
- ½ cup pineapple
- 2 teaspoons honey

Directions:
1. Add listed ingredients to a blender
2. Blend until you have a smooth and creamy texture
3. Serve chilled and enjoy!

Nutrition Info: Calories: 324; Fat: 25.4g; Carbohydrates: 18g; Protein: 4.3g

Cherry-berry Smoothie

Servings: 2
Cooking Time: 2 Minutes
Ingredients:
- ¾ cup sweet or sour cherries (fresh or frozen)
- ¼ cup blueberries (fresh or frozen)
- ½ cup unsweetened almond milk
- 1 cup plain Greek yogurt
- 1 large banana, chopped (fresh or frozen)
- ½ teaspoon vanilla extract
- 3-4 ice cubes

Directions:
1. Add everything to your blender and pulse it on high for 20 seconds and your smoothie is ready. Enjoy!

Nutrition Info: (Per Serving): Calories- 105, Fat- 1.2 g, Protein- 5.1 g, Carbohydrates-22 g

Cacao – Avocado Smoothie

Servings: 1 Large
Cooking Time: 2 Minutes
Ingredients:
- 1 cup organic coconut milk
- 4 teaspoons cacao powder
- ½ avocado, peeled, pitted and chopped
- 4-5 drops liquid Stevia (optional)
- 1 teaspoon Chia seeds
- 4-5 ice cubes

Directions:
1. Add everything into the blender jar and process until nice and thick.

Nutrition Info: (Per Serving): Calories- 285, Fat- 23 g, Protein- 8 g, Carbohydrates- 23 g

Strawberry – Banana Smoothie

Servings: 2
Cooking Time: 5 Minutes
Ingredients:
- 2 small heads of bok choy
- 2 cups whole strawberries (fresh or frozen)
- 1 large banana, chopped (fresh or frozen)
- 2 tablespoon avocado flesh
- 1 teaspoon flax seed powder
- ½ cup filtered water

Directions:
1. Combine all the ingredients in the blender and pulse until smooth

Nutrition Info: (Per Serving): Calories- 290, Fat- 10 g, Protein- 6.2 g, Carbohydrates- 55 g

Appendix : Recipes Index

Oats And Berry Smoothie 38
3 Spice-almond Smoothie 90
4 Superfood Spice Smoothie 52

A

A Batch Of Slimming Berries 46
A Green Grape Shake 50
A Honeydew And Cucumber Medley 50
A Mean Green Milk Shake 78
A Melon Cucumber Medley 14
A Peachy Perfect Glass 48
A Whole Melon Surprise 87
A-b-c Smoothie 25
Acai Berry And Orange Smoothie 54
All In 1 Smoothie 93
Almond And Choco-brownie Shake 21
Almond And Date Smoothie 60
Almond- Citrus Punch 35
Almond- Melon Punch 35
Almond-banana Blend 36
Almond-banana Booster 96
Aloe Berry Smoothie 95
Aloe Vera Smoothie 72
Apple Berry Smoothie 30
Apple Blackberry Wonder 43
Apple- Blueberry Smoothie 91
Apple Celery Detox Smoothie 17
Apple Chia Detox Smoothie 58
Apple Cucumber 42
Apple- Date Smoothie 98
Apple Kale Krusher 55
Apple –kiwi Blush 69
Apple Mango Cucumber Crush 21
Apple, Carrot, Ginger & Fennel Smoothie 84
Apple, Dried Figs And Lemon Smoothie 45
Apple, Strawberry & Beet Smoothie 63
Apple-beet Smoothie 16
Apple-kiwi Slush 7
Apple papaya Medley 86
Avocado And Blueberry Smoothie 82
Avocado And Edamame Drink 105
Avocado- Citrus Blast 41
Avocado Detox Smoothie 15
Avocado Turmeric Smoothie 103
Avocado Wonder Smoothie 96
Awesome Pineapple And Carrot Blend 98

B

Banana And Spinach Raspberry Smoothie 24
Banana Apple Blast 99
Banana- Cantaloupe Wonder 45
Banana Green Smoothie 76
Banana- Guava Smoothie 68
Banana Oatmeal Detox Smoothie 56
Banana Orange Pina Colada 47
Banana, Almond, And Dark Chocolate Smoothie 26
Banana-avocado Smoothie 9
Banana-beet Smoothie 38
Banana-cado Smoothie 30
Banana-mango Delight 26
Banana-sunflower Coconut Smoothie 75
Basic Green Banana Smoothie 58
Basil- Bee Pollen Chlorella Smoothie 72
Beet And Apple Smoothie 38
Beet And Grapefruit Smoothie 83
Beet And Pineapple Smoothie 57
Beet Berry Chiller 34
Beets And Berry Beauty Enhancer 50
Berrilicious Chiller 9
Berry Banana Smoothie 35
Berry Beautiful Glowing Skin Smoothie 95
Berry Berry Smoothie 87
Berry Carrot Smoothie 8
Berry Collard Green Smoothie 78
Berry Dessert Smoothie 92
Berry Dreamsicle Smoothie 22
Berry Flax Smoothie 97
Berry- Green Tea Fusion Smoothie 88
Berry Infusion Smoothie 89
Berry Melon Green Smoothie 72
Berry- Mint Cooler 101
Berry Mint Smoothie 10
Berry Orange Madness 20
Berry Peachy Blush 31
Berry Spinach Basil Smoothie 76
Berry Truffle Smoothie 105
Berry-banana-spinach Smoothie 28
Berry-beet Watermelon Smoothie 45
Berry-cantaloupe Smoothie 70
Berry-licious Meta Booster 104
Berry-ssimon Carrot Smoothie 41
Blackberry Green Smoothie 80
Blackberry Mango Crunch 73
Bluberry Cucumber Cooler 92
Blue And Green Wonder 75
Blue Dragon Smoothie 41
Blueberry & Cucumber Smoothie 66
Blueberry Cherry Wellness Potion 42
Blueberry Chia Smoothie 58
Blueberry Detox Drink 14
Blueberry Peach Smoothie 8
Blueberry Pineapple Blast Smoothie 33
Blueberry–avocado Smoothie 26
Brain Nutrition-analyzer 91
Bright Rainbow Health 87

C

Cacao – Avocado Smoothie 106
Cacao Cantaloupe Smoothie 16
Cacao- Goji Berry Almond Smoothie 54
Cacao Mango Green Smoothie 80
Cacao- Spirulina And Berry Booster 10

Cacao-goji Berry Marvel 90
Cantaloupe Berry Blast 47
Cantaloupe Yogurt Smoothie 95
Caramel Banana Smoothie 84
Carrot And Prune Crunch 59
Carrot Crunch Smoothie 74
Carrot Detox Smoothie 14
Carrot Peach Blush 33
Carrot Spice Smoothie 28
Carrot, Watermelon And Cumin Smoothie 49
Cashew Apple Glass 102
Cashew- Goji Berry Smoothie 105
Cauliflower Cold Glass 48
Chai Coconut Shake 46
Chai Tea Smoothie 84
Charcoal Lemonade Detox Smoothie 15
Chard, Lime & Mint Smoothies 85
Cheery Charlie Checker 90
Cherry & Beet Smoothie 64
Cherry & Blueberry Smoothie 62
Cherry & Kale Smoothie 63
Cherry & Pineapple Smoothie 62
Cherry Acai Berry Smoothie 81
Cherry- Date Plum Smoothie 40
Cherry-berry Smoothie 106
Cherry-vanilla Smoothie 29
Chia And Cherry Smoothie 63
Chia Berry Cucumber Smoothie 17
Chia Berry Spinach Smoothie 73
Chia Flax Berry Green Smoothie 75
Chia Mango-nut Smoothie 44
Chia, Blueberry & Banana Smoothie 82
Chia-blueberry Smoothie 24
Chia-cacao Melon Smoothie 35
Chilled Watermelon Krush 31
Choco- Berry Delight 74
Chocolate Shake Smoothie 93
Chocolate Spinach Smoothie 33
Chocolaty Berry Blast 94
Cilantro And Citrus Glass 81
Cilantro- Grapefriut Smoothie 70
Cilantro-lemon Smoothie 13
Cinna-melon Detox Smoothie 15
Cinnammon-apple Green Smoothie 91
Cinnamon Mango Smoothie 99
Cinn-apple Beet Smoothie 36
Citrus Coconut Punch 41
Citrus Green Smoothie 77
Citrus Spinach Immune Booster 11
Clementine Green Smoothie 76
Clemintine Dreamsicle Smoothie 27
Coco- Cranberry Smoothie 99
Cocoa Banana Smoothie 33
Cocoa Pumpkin 12
Coco-banann Green Smoothie 81
Coco-maca Smoothie 9
Coco-nana Smoothie 100

Coconut Berry Smoothie 60
Coconut Blue Wonder 74
Coconut Carrot Pleasure 65
Coconut- Flaxseed Smoothie 100
Coconut -mint Smoothie 106
Coconut Mulberry Banana Smoothie 53
Coconut Peach Passion 18
Coconut Pear Crunch Smoothie 103
Coconut Pineapple Detox Smoothie 16
Coconut Strawberry Punch 33
Coconut-banana Smoothie 97
Coconut-blueberry Smoothie 71
Coconutty Apple Smoothie 27
Cool Coco-loco Cream Shake 32
Cool Strawberry 365 56
Creamy Pink Smoothie 10
Crunchy Kale – Chia Smoothie 94
Cucumber Kale And Lime Apple Smoothie 27
Cucumber Kiwi Crush 90
Cucumber- Pear Healer 70
Cucumber- Pineapple 70
Cucumber-kale Chiller 103

D

Dandelion And Carrot Booster 98
Dandellion Green Berry Smoothie 78
Dandellion- Orange Smoothie 12
Dark Chocolate Peppermint Smoothie 23
Date "n" Banana Smoothie 42
Date And Apricot Green Smoothie 79
Date And Walnut Wonder 54
Date Pomegranate Wonder 30
Delicious Creamy Choco Shake 34
Delish Pineapple And Coconut Milk Smoothie 32
Diabetic Berry Blast 104
Double Decker Smoothie 7
Dragon- Berry Smoothie 40
Dragon Fruit And Beet Smoothie 54
Drink Your Salad Smoothie 43

E

Electrifying Green Smoothie 77

F

Finana Smoothie 43
Fine Tea Toner 51
Fine Yo "mama" Matcha 59
Flax And Almond Butter Smoothie 25
Flax And Kiwi Spinach Smoothie 27
Flaxseed And Berry Smoothie 8
Fruit "n" Nut Smoothie 69
Fruit Bomb Smoothie 40

G

Garden Variety Green And Yogurt Delight 77
Generous Mango Surprise 99
Ginger Banana Kick 35
Ginger Cantaloupe Detox Smoothie 45
Ginger Lime Smoothie 69
Ginger- Papaya Smoothie 68

Ginger- Parsely Grape Smoothie 68
Ginger Plum Punch 20
Ginger- Pomegranate Smoothie 97
Ginger-carrot Punch 65
Ginger-mango Berry Blush 47
Glorious Cinnamon Roll Smoothie 22
Goji Berry- Pineapple Wonder 98
Grape And Nectarine Blende 61
Grape And Spinach Smoothie 28
Grape And Strawberry Smoothie 94
Grapefruit Spinach Smoothie 86
Great Green Garden 61
Great Nutty Lion 89
Green Chia Smoothie 73
Green Goblin Smoothie 64
Green Grapefruit Smoothie 17
Green Protein Smoothie 20
Green Skinny Energizer 96
Green Smoothie 83
Green Tea And Carrot Smoothie 102
Green Tea- Berry Smoothie 13
Green Tea- Mango Smoothie 29
Green Tea Superfood Smooothie 73
Green Tea-cacao Berry Smoothie 52
Greenie Genie S Moothie 78
Greens And Herbs For All 104
Guava Berry Smoothie 62

H
Hale 'n' Kale Banana Smoothie 88
Healthy Chocolate Milkshake 23
Healthy Kiwi Smoothie 83
Healthy Potato Pie Glass 102
Healthy Raspberry And Coconut Glass 24
Hearty Cucumber Quencher 16
Hearty Papaya Drink 60
Hemp And Kale Smoothie 102
Hemp, Date And Chia Smoothie 74
Hemp-avocado Smoothie 38
Honey And Cacao Bliss Smoothie 20
Honeydewmelon And Mint Blast 14

I
Iron And Protein Shake 19

K
Kale & Avocado Smoothie 64
Kale And Pomegranate Smoothie 93
Kale Celery Smoothie 29
Kale, Cucumber Cooler 31
Keto Mocha Smoothie 105
Kiwi- Banana Healer 8
Kiwi Cooler 10
Kiwi Quick Smoothie 69
Kiwi-berry-nana 38

L
Leeks And Broccoli Cucumber Glass 24
Lemon Cilantro Delight 80
Lettuce -0range Cooler 49
Lime & Green Tea Smoothie Bowl 82
Lime "n" Lemony Cucumber Cooler 104
Lime And Lemon Detox Punch 12
Lime And Melon Healer 35
Lovely Green Gazpacho 77
Lychee- Cucumber Cooler 55
Lychee Green Smoothie 40

M
Maca – Mango Delight 51
Maca- Almond Protein Smoothie Shake 22
Maca –banana Smoothie 71
Mad Mocha Glass 20
Mang0-soy Smoothie 89
Mango And Blueberry Bean Smoothie 54
Mango Beet Energy Booster 101
Mango Cantaloupe Smoothie 43
Mango- Chia- Coconut Smoothie 86
Mango Delight 18
Mango Energizer 101
Mango Grape Smoothie 77
Mango Honey Smoothie 97
Mango Mania 23
Mango- Papaya Blend 64
Mango Passion Smoothie 47
Mango Smoothie 85
Mango Strawberry Smoothie 28
Mango, Lime & Spinach Smoothie 83
Mango-almond Smoothie 56
Mango-berry Smoothie 47
Mango-cado Blush 93
Mango-ginger Tango 37
Mango-pina Smoothie 65
Matcha Coconut Smoothie 87
Mct Strawberry Smoothie 100
Meanie-greenie Weigh Loss Smoothie 27
Melon And Soy Smoothie 36
Melon-berry And Ginger Smoothie 12
Mesmerizing Strawberry And Chocolate Shake 32
Mini Pepper Popper Smoothie 49
Mint And Avocado Smoothie 36
Mint And Kale Smoothie 25
Min-tea Mango Rejuvinating Smoothie 92
Mint-pineapple Cooler 60
Minty Cantaloupe Smoothie 79
Mixed- Berry Wonder 88
Mixed Fruit Madness 30
Mixed Fruit Magic Smoothie 8
Mp3 Smoothie 42
Multi-berry Smoothie 7

N
Natural Nectarine 55
Noteworthy Vitamin C 57
Nutty Apple Smoothie 44
Nutty Bean "n"berry Smoothie 89
Nutty Mango Green Blend 74
Nutty Raspberry Avocado Blend 95

O

Oat And Walnut Berry Blast 73
Oat, Celery Green Smoothie 104
Oatmeal Banana Smoothie 37
Oats And Blueberry Smoothie 98
Orange Antioxidant Refresher 96
Orange Banana Smoothie 48
Orange- Broccoli Green Monster 87
Orange Coco Smoothie 10
Orange Cranberry Smoothie 43
Orange Gold Smoothie 70
Orange- Green Tonic 94
Orange Kiwi Punch 68
Orange Squash Tango 63
Orange Sunrise Smoothie 68

P

Papaya Berry Banana Blend 17
Papaya- Mint Chiller 59
Papaya Passion 7
Passion Green Smoothie 76
Peach And Celery Smoothie 37
Peach-ban-illa Smoothie 36
Peachy Ginger Smoothie 66
Peachyfig Green Smoothie 44
Peanut Butter And Raspberry Delight 105
Peanut Butter Broccoli Smoothie 30
Peanut Butter Chocolate Protein Shake 19
Peanut Butter Jelly Smoothie 34
Peanut Butter, Banana And Cacao Smoothie 27
Pear 'n' Kale Smoothie 86
Pear And Avocado Smoothie 57
Pear Jicama Detox Smoothie 13
Pear, Peach & Papaya Smoothie 66
Pear-simmon Smoothie 40
Peppermint And Dark Chocolate Shake Delight 19
Peppermint Stick Smoothie 100
Persimmon Pineapple Protein Smoothie 96
Pina Berry Smoothie 38
Pina Colada Smoothie 83
Pina-banana And Grapefruit Smoothie 64
Pineapple & Almond Smoothie 62
Pineapple & Coconut Smoothie 62
Pineapple & Green Tea Smoothie 66
Pineapple & Mango Smoothie 62
Pineapple & Watermelon Smoothie 65
Pineapple And Cucumber Cooler 81
Pineapple Banana Smoothie 30
Pineapple Basil Blast 53
Pineapple Broccoli Smoothie 106
Pineapple Coconut Detox Smoothie 14
Pineapple- Flax Smoothie 56
Pineapple Papaya Perfection Smoothie 31
Pineapple Protein Smoothie 22
Pineapple Sage Smoothie 70
Pineapple Yogurt Smoothie 58
Pineapple, Mango & Coconut Smoothie 63
Pineapple-pear And Spinach Smoothie 37
Pink Grapefruit Skin 93
Pink Potion 94
Plum- Bokchoy Smoothie 102
Pomegranate- Berry Smoothie 11
Pomegranate- Ginger Melba 46
Pomegranate, Tangerine And Ginger Smoothie 89
Popoye's Pear Smoothie For Kids 8
Powerful Green Frenzy 97
Powerful Kale And Carrot Glass 50
Powerful Purple Smoothie 100
Protein-packed Root Beer Shake 21
Pumpkin- Banana Spicy Delight 47
Pumpkin Pie Buttered Coffee 26
Pumpkin Power Smoothie 99
Pumpkin Spice Smoothie 93
Punchy Watermelon 16
Punpkin Seed And Yogurt Smoothie 96

Q

Quick Berry Banana Smoothie 48

R

Raspberry And White Chocolate Shake 21
Raspberry Carrot Smoothie 72
Raspberry- Grapefruit Smoothie 26
Raspberry Peach Delight 74
Raspberry Pecan Date Delight 33
Raspberry Smoothie 84
Rasp-ricot Smoothie 40
Raw Chocolate Smoothie 32
Red Healing Potion 42
Rosemary And Lemon Garden Smoothie 86

S

Saffron Oats Smoothie 92
Sage Blackberry 46
Sapodilla, Chia And Almond Milk Smoothie 59
Simple Anti-aging Cacao Dream 51
Slim-jim Vanilla Latte 48
Snicker Doodle Smoothie 21
Spiced Banana Smoothie 65
Spiced Pineapple Smoothie 25
Spiced Up Banana Shake 18
Spicy Pear And Green Tea 103
Spin-a-banana Smoothie 59
Spinach And Grape Smoothie 36
Spinach And Kiwi Smoothie 69
Spinach, Carrot And Tomato Smoothie 24
Spinach, Grape, & Coconut Smoothie 82
Spin-a-mango Green Protein Smoothie 19
Spin-apple Pear Smoothie 57
Straight Up Avocado And Kale Smoothie 25
Strawberry – Banana Smoothie 106
Strawberry & Kale Smoothie 65
Strawberry Coconut Snowflake 18
Strawberry Watermelon Smoothie 84
Strawberry-avocado Smoothie 68
Strawberry-chia Smoothie 39
Strawberry-ginger Tea Smoothie 9

Subtle Raspberry Smoothie 22
Super Avocado Smoothie 82
Super Duper Berry Smoothie 55
Super Tropi-kale Wonder 75
Super-detox Smoothie 14
Sweet And Spicy Fruit Punch 66
Sweet Pea Smoothie 90
Sweet Potato & Orange Smoothie 67
Sweet Protein And Cherry Shake 18

T

Tangerine- Ginger Flu Busting Smoothie 9
Tangy Mango & Spinach Smoothie 63
Tea And Grape Smoothie 72
The Amazing Acai 61
The Anti-aging Avocado 52
The Anti-aging Superfood Glass 52
The Anti-aging Turmeric And Coconut Delight 50
The Baked Apple 56
The Big Blue Delight 46
The Big Bomb Pop 49
The Blueberry Bliss 88
The Breezy Blueberry 53
The Cacao Super Smoothie 18
The Coolest 5 Lettuce Green Shake 76
The Curious Raspberry And Green Shake 76
The Deep Green Lagoon 79
The Feisty Goddess 51
The Glass Of Glowing Skin 52
The Great Avocado And Almond Delight 19
The Great Shamrock Shake 45
The Green Potato Chai 80
The Gritty Coffee Shake 86
The Minty Cucumber 79
The Nutty Macadamia Delight 60
The Overloaded Berry Shake 31
The Pinky Swear 45
The Pumpkin Eye 57
The Super Green 53
The Wild Matcha Delight 78
The Wisest Watermelon Glass 89
The Wrinkle Fighter 51
Tomato- Melon Refreshing Smoothie 60
Trimelon Melba 43
Triple Berry Delight 105
Tropical Apple Coconut Green Blend 80
Tropical Greens Smoothie 88
Tropical Kiwi Pineapple 103
Tropical Matcha Kale 77
Tropical Smoothie 15
Tropical Storm Glass 57
Twisty Cucumber Honeydew 12

U

Ultimate Berry Blush 32
Ultimate Cold And Flu Fighting Smoothie 11
Ultimate Orange Potion 54
Ultimate Super Food Smoothie 92

V

Vanilla- Mango Madness 37
Veggie Wonder 28
Verry- Berry Breakfast 98
Verry-berry Carrot Delight 39
Very Berry Blueberry Wonder 32
Very Creamy Green Machine 21
Very-berry Orange 13
Vitamin-c Boost Smoothie 7

W

Water-mato Green Smoothie 41
Watermelon- Yogurt Smoothie 53
Watermelon, Berries & Avocado Smoothie 64
Wheatgrass Detox Smoothie 15

Y

Yogi- Banana Agave Smoothie 41
Yogi-berry Smoothie 11
Yogurt And Plum Smoothie 58

Z

Zucchini Apple Smoothie 25
Zucchini Detox Smoothie 13

Lightning Source UK Ltd.
Milton Keynes UK
UKHW030630051022
409964UK00013B/1135